MANUAL OF CHILD DEVE

Already published

Paediatric Gastroenterology *J. H. Tripp and D. C. A. Candy*
Renal Disease *C. B. Brown*
Haematology *A. S. J. Baughan, A. S. B. Hughes, K. G. Patterson and
L. Stirling*
Clinical Blood Transfusion *B. Brozovic and M. Brozovic*
Chest Medicine *J. E. Stark, J. M. Shneerson, T. Higenbottam and
C. D. R. Flower*
Gynaecology *T. R. Varma*
Cardiology *K. Dawkins*
Rheumatology *J. M. H. Moll*
Hospital Paediatrics *G. Hambleton*
Gastroenterology *B. T. Cooper and R. E. Berry*

Forthcoming volumes in the Manuals series

Neonatal Medicine *D. R. Harvey and M. Cummins*
Geriatric Medicine *A. N. Exton-Smith and T. Van der Cammen*

MANUAL OF CHILD DEVELOPMENT

Sundara Lingam MD (Hons) MRCP DRCOG DCH

Consultant Paediatrician with special interest in Community Child Health,
Princess Alexandra Hospital, Essex

David R Harvey FRCP DCH

Consultant Paediatrician, Queen Charlotte's
Hospital for Women, London

Churchill Livingstone

EDINBURGH LONDON MELBOURNE AND NEW YORK 1988

CHURCHILL LIVINGSTONE
Medical Division of Longman Group UK Limited

Distributed in the United States of America by
Churchill Livingstone Inc., 1560 Broadway, New York,
N. Y. 10036, and by associated companies, branches
and representatives throughout the world.

First published 1991

ISBN 0-443-04593-3

British Library Cataloguing in Publication Data

Lingam, Sundara
    Manual of child development.
    1. Child development—Testing
    I. Title   II. Harvey, David R.
    155.4   RJ131

Library of Congress Cataloging in Publication Data

Lingam, Sundara, 1944–
    Manual of child development.

    (Manuals series)
    Includes index.
    1. Child development—Handbooks, manuals, etc.
2. Children—Medical examinations—Handbooks, manuals,
etc. I. Harvey, David (David Robert) II. Title
[DNLM: 1. Child Development—handbooks. 2. Child
Development Disorders—diagnosis—handbooks. 3. Physical
Examination in infancy & childhood—handbooks.
WS 39 L755m]
RJ131.L54 1987   618.92'075   87–15861

Printed in Great Britain at The Bath Press, Avon

PREFACE

The intention of this pocket-book is to provide short notes on the basic developmental screening techniques used for children between the ages of 6 weeks and 5 years. Health visitors and others concerned with child development have told us that they need such a manual for use in practice and for teaching. We therefore hope this book will be useful to all those working in the community health services. Developmental screening will be done increasingly by members of the primary care team. More and more general practitioners are undertaking child health surveillance, and health visitors are doing many of the tests. These screening tests are not only important in reassuring doctors, health visitors and parents that the child's development is proceeding within normal limits, but the consultations also give parents the chance to discuss minor problems that may be worrying them.

Changes in undergraduate paediatric teaching and in higher medical examinations (MRCP and DCH) have placed greater emphasis on developmental screening methods. The Royal Colleges of Physicians of the United Kingdom have recommended that all MRCP candidates should be examined in developmental screening, while the DCH examination has given greater prominence to community paediatrics and developmental screening. Candidates in these examinations are of course expected to test vision and hearing. This book will thus be useful for undergraduate and postgraduate students; it will also be of use as a manual for clinical medical officers and should serve as a guide during their child health clinic sessions.

ACKNOWLEDGEMENTS

The scheme described in this book has been brought together from a number of original sources. It is a pleasure to acknowledge the pioneering work of Mary Sheridan, Dorothy Egan and the team who produced the Denver Developmental Screening Test. We also would like to thank Dr John Wilson and Dr Ann Brown for their helpful comments on the Developmental Chart, and Cow and Gate Limited for producing the chart as a service to promote better child care.

The drawings are by Oëna Armstrong and the manuscript was prepared with help from Susan Reid, Director of Publications, Success Tutors.

CONTENTS

1 INTRODUCTION

DEVELOPMENTAL SCREENING

Developmental screening is only a part of child health surveillance, which includes general health education, immunisation and specific advice on nutrition and safety. The screening programme is aimed at providing pre-symptomatic detection of disability by examining children serially to determine whether they are developing normally. It is carried out on apparently healthy children and takes into account the ages at which they achieve skills. The intention is to discover developmental delay or behaviour problems as early as possible, because many causes of slow development, for example a hearing deficit or psychosocial deprivation, may be treated with satisfactory results if detected early enough.

The screening programme is devised for the secondary and tertiary prevention of disability. Secondary prevention is the early detection of disease before symptoms or disordered function appear and when appropriate action may stop or reverse the disease process. Tertiary prevention is the management of established disease to avoid or limit the development of a disability and its subsequent handicap. (Primary prevention is prevention by removing the cause of handicap.)

The screening procedure should be brief, simple, cheap and reliable, so that it can be carried out on large numbers of children. Our personal preference for screening times is when the child is 6 weeks, 8 months, 18 months, 2½ and 4–5 years of age. The screening may be combined with visits for immunisation, but the developmental screening tests should be done first.

In the UK, screening is carried out by a doctor or health visitor. At present, the policy differs from district to district. It may be done at child health clinics (community health service clinics) by clinical medical officers or by general practitioners interested in developmental screening, at their surgeries. However, in developing countries it may be performed by trained non-professionals.

At some of the consultations for developmental screening it is essential to perform a general medical examination, including abduction of the hips, palpation of the testes, auscultation of the heart and examination of the eyes for squint.

It is important that anyone undertaking screening should have a clear idea of what is normal or abnormal, and that there is a quick and practical line of referral. A test is not satisfactory if there is no clear answer and if referral means a waiting time of several months before development assessment. A child who passes all screening tests is not necessarily normal — he may develop or manifest a disability later.

It should be noted that *developmental screening* is not the same as *developmental assessment* which is a more detailed examination to elucidate the underlying problem and to make a diagnosis.

Practical point   If a child fails a screening test, ask the parents, health visitor or nursery group for their opinion. Re-examine 1 month later to confirm the finding and, if the child still fails, refer him for developmental assessment. Do not say to parents immediately: 'Looks to me as though there is some deviation from what is expected of . . .; I think it may be best to arrange for a full assessment'.

DEVELOPMENTAL ASSESSMENT

Developmental assessment is carried out on a child discovered by developmental screening to have developmental delay or behaviour disorder, to establish whether there is a problem and, if so, the type and causes. Its aim is to plan management, including treatment and genetic counselling, and to advise parents on how to cope and live with a handicapped child. An individual plan of management should be provided.

The assessment is performed by a team (District Child Development Team) led by a developmental paediatrician or consultant paediatrician in community child health. It includes assessment by a physiotherapist, a speech therapist, an occupational therapist and often by a psychologist as well.

Developmental assessment is a time-consuming procedure which may take several days to complete. It does *not* predict the future; it only assesses what the child can do at the time of assessment.

PHYSICAL EXAMINATION

Physical examination should be undertaken at each developmental screening examination, but it is not part of the screening itself. Equipment required for the examination is a stethoscope, ophthalmoscope, auriscope, sphygmomanometer, tendon hammer, spatula and tape measure; and access to a weighing scale is necessary.

Particular importance should be given to the following.

1 *Dysmorphic features*. These are minor congenital abnormalities which may occur in the normal population. If there are several in the same child, this suggests that a recognisable syndrome may be present.

2 *Height, weight and head circumference*. These should be plotted on centile charts.

3 *Blood pressure*. This should be taken routinely in children over 4 years of age.

Not every child needs to be examined with the auriscope or the ophthalmoscope. If the hearing is suspect, check the ears for wax and note the state of the tympanic membrane; if the vision is suspect, check for cataract, choroiditis and retrolental fibroplasia and examine the optic discs.

Note   Physical and neurological examination may give a clue to the problem of development, e.g. Down's syndrome, hypothyroidism, mucopolysaccharidoses.

Examine both parents as they may have the same abnormality, e.g. dysmorphic features, or a large or small head.

Tone is an important neurological sign. Increased tone in the limbs is often significant. Check for this carefully at 6–8 months, as it may be an early sign of spasticity. A child with hypotonia should also be carefully followed, as this may be due to a neuromuscular problem, although sometimes it is benign.

SCREENING FOR THE VARIOUS ASPECTS OF DEVELOPMENT

Four aspects of development are checked: (a) gross motor; (b) fine motor and vision; (c) hearing and speech; (d) social behaviour and play.

The screening is performed to find out what the child can do, not what he cannot do. This is why the history is important because young children often do things at home which they refuse to do in strange surroundings, such as a clinic. However, in some tests which are passed by examination the child's performance must be observed. In the text on the following pages, normal ranges have been included where these are known.

Development is observed in each of the four aspects. A child who is slow in all four is likely to have mental retardation, provided emotional and social deprivation have been excluded. A child with normal gross and fine development, without abnormality in vision, social behaviour and play, but with delayed language development, is unlikely to have mental retardation. His problem is probably isolated language delay. Similarly, a child who only has delay in walking is unlikely to have intellectual impairment.

GRQSS MOTOR

Gross motor concerns posture and large movements, especially walking and balance; it also includes head control, sitting, throwing and catching.

FINE MOTOR AND VISION

Fine motor deals with hand manipulation, reaching and grasping; vision deals with sight. Both together deal with hand–eye co-ordination, finger control and the placing and replacing of objects.

HEARING AND SPEECH

Normal hearing is necessary for speech and language development; tests for hearing and language development are included in this section. Language development concerns the comprehension and expression of language.

Note   Speech and language development is greatly influenced by the environment.

SOCIAL BEHAVIOUR AND PLAY

Play helps children to learn. It concerns social and personal relationships, such as interaction with other children and with adults, the show of affection and the child's understanding of games, order and tidiness.

In addition, play is important for self-care (such as dressing, feeding, toilet training and table manners and with the development of individual personality). It also concerns adaptive development problem-solving skills and adaptability to objects and situations.

Note   Social development is greatly influenced by cultural customs.

MATERIALS REQUIRED FOR DEVELOPMENTAL SCREENING

The following are a list of items which have proved invaluable in developmental screening:

1 A bright object, e.g. a red woollen ball — this may easily be made.
2 Manchester and Nuffield rattles or similar rattles (available from Stycar*).
3 Cup and spoon.
4 Bell.
5 Twelve 2½ cm (1 inch) square bricks in four colour — red, blue, yellow and green.
6 Beads and stick.
7 Pencil and paper.
8 Small objects: raisins, Smarties (small coloured sweets) and cake decorations such as 'hundreds and thousands' and 'silver balls'.
9 Toys for the speech discrimination test (see page 48).

*A 'Developkit', which includes most materials required for screening tests, is in preparation (available from Success Tutors, Shop 4, Second Avenue, East Vale, Acton, London W3 7RU).

2 CHILD DEVELOPMENT

NORMAL MILESTONES

DEVELOPMENTAL SCREENING

For some items the approximate range when 25–90% of normal children can do the test (pass) is given, mainly using data from the Denver Developmental Screening Test.

6 weeks old

Gross motor	Head control (0–3 months) Moro response* Ventral suspension (0–1 month) Prone position*
Fine motor and vision	Stares* Follows horizontally to 90°
Hearing and speech	Rattle or bell 15 cm at ear level* Startle response*
Social behaviour	Smiles (0–10 weeks, mean 5 weeks) Turns to regard observer's face*
Warning signs at 6 weeks	No visual fixation or following Failure to respond to sound Asymmetrical neonatal reflexes Excessive head leg Failure to smile

*Should be present at birth (term).

Note   Allow for pre-term birth (age = corrected age).

6–8 months old

Gross motor	Bears weight on legs (3–7 months) Downward parachute response (4–6 months) Sits with support (4–6 months) Sits without support (5–8) months) Can be pulled to sit (3½–6 months) Forward parachute response (7–10 months) Crawls (6–9 months)
Fine motor and vision	Reaches out to grasp (palmer grasp) (3–6 months) Transfers and mouths (4½–8 months) Fixes on small objects (5–8 months) Follows fallen toys or red woollen ball (4½–8 months)
Hearing and speech	Vocalises (4–6 months) Polysyllabic babbling (6–10 months) Laughs (2–5 months) Responds to own name (4–8 months) Distraction hearing test*
Social behaviour and play	Puts everything to mouth (4–8 months) Hand and foot regard (4–8 months) Plays peek-a-boo (5½–10 months)
Warning signs at 8 months	Hand preference, fisting, squint Persistence of primitive reflexes — Moro response, stepping, and the asymmetrical tonic neck reflex.

*Many babies will not respond well at 6 months; this test is best deferred to 8–10 months.

12 months old

Gross motor	Gets to sitting position (6–11 months) Pulls to standing position (6–10 months) Walks holding furniture (7–13 months) Walks alone (10–15 months)
Fine motor and vision	Points with index finger Casts (throws) (9–15 months) Pincer grasp (9–14 months) Holds 2 bricks and bangs them together (7–13 months)
Hearing and speech	Turns to sound of name Uses 'mama' and 'dada' (11–20 months; 50% children by 15 months) Understands several words Distraction hearing test
Social behaviour and play	Drinks from cup (10–16 months) Indicates wants (not by crying) (10–15 months) Play 'pat-a-cake' (8–13 months) Waves good-bye (8–13 months)
Warning signs at 12 months	Unable to sit or bear weight (except in congenital hypotonia, when delayed motor development is usual) Persistence of hand regard Absence of babbling and cooing Absence of saving reactions

Note   Allow for pre-term birth (age = corrected age).

18 months old

Gross motor	Walks backwards (12–22 months) Carries toys while walking Climbs stairs (14–22 months) Climbs onto chair
Fine motor and vision	Delicate pincer grasp (10–18 months) Scribbles (12–24 months) Turns páges Builds tower of 3 or 4 bricks (16–24 months)

Hearing and speech	Jabbers continually
	Utters 3 or more words other than 'mama' and 'dada'
	    (10–21 months)
	Points to eyes, nose and mouth (14–23 months)
	Obeys simple instructions — 'close the door'
	    (15 months–2½ years)*

Social behaviour and play	Holds spoon: gets food to mouth (14 months–2½ years) Explores environment (13–20 months) Takes off shoes and socks (13–20 months) Indicates toilet needs

Warning signs at 18 months	Inability to stand without support
	    (NB Children who shuffle on bottom walk late —
	    mean age 22 months)
	Inability to understand simple commands
	No spontaneous vocalisation
	No pincer grip
	Casting (throwing) still present

*By 12 months, 50% of normal children can speak 6–10 words with meaning and, by 21 months, 97%.

2½ years old

Gross motor	Climbs and descends stairs Jumps in place (21 months–3 years) Kicks ball (15–24 months)
Fine motor and vision	Picks up 'hundreds and thousands' Imitates vertical line (18 months–2 years 9 months) Builds tower of 8 bricks (21 months–3 years 6 months)
Hearing and speech	Uses plurals (20 months–3 years 3 months) Gives name Hearing test*; speech discrimination test
Social behaviour and play	Plays alone Eats with spoon and fork Puts on clothes Dry throughout day
Warning signs at 2½ years	Unable to speak in short sentences[1] Unable to understand speech (differentiate from understanding situations by visual clues)

*May co-operate for audiometry; if hearing is suspect do not delay audiological assessment.
[1]By 23 months, 50% of normal children can join words into simple sentences and, by 3 years, 97%.
Girls are slightly more advanced than boys.

3 years old

Gross motor	Runs fast Climbs stairs in adult manner Pedals tricycle (21 months–3 years) Stands on one foot for 1 second (22 months–3 years 3 months)
Fine motor and vision	Copies circle (2 years 3 months–3 years 6 months) Threads beads well Matches 2 colours
Hearing and speech	Uses prepositions (3 years–4 years 6 months) Uses sentences of 4 words* Gives full name, sex and age (2 years 6 months–4 years)
Social behaviour and play	Eats with knife and fork Goes to toilet alone Dresses with supervision (2 years 3 months–3 years 6 months) Washes and dries hands (20 months–3 years 3 months) Separates from mother easily (2–4 years)

*See warning signs at 2½ years.

4 years old*

Gross motor	Hops on one foot for 2 metres forward (3–5 years) Climbs ladder/tree/slide Stands on one foot for 5 seconds (2 years 9 months–4 years 6 months) Walks heel-to-toe (3 years 6 months–5 years 3 months)
Fine motor and vision	Copies cross and square[1] Imitates bridge of 3 bricks Draws man with 3 parts
Hearing and speech	Speaks grammatically (2 years 7 months–4 years 2 months) Counts up to 10 Gives full name, age and address Recognises colours (3 years–4 years 9 months)
Social behaviour and play	Shares toys Brushes teeth Dresses without supervision (3 years 4 months–5 years 6 months)
Warning signs	Speech difficult to understand because of poor articulation, or because of omission or substitution of consonants.

*May co-operate for audiometry; if hearing is suspect do not delay audiological assessment.
[1]Copies cross (3–4½ years); copies square (4–5½ years).

5 years old

Gross motor	Walks downstairs one foot per step Bounces and catches ball (3 years 3 months–5 years 6 months) Walks backwards heel-to-toe (4 years–6 years)
Fine motor and vision	Copies triangle (5 years 6 months) Draws men with all features (4 years 6 months–6 years) Copies 3 steps from 6 bricks
Hearing and speech	Speaks fluently and clearly* Hearing test—audiometry
Social behaviour and play	Comforts friends in distress Chooses own friends Dramatic group play

*Confusion of 's', 'f' and 'th' (disappears by 6½ years).

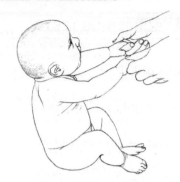

Fig. 1 Head control

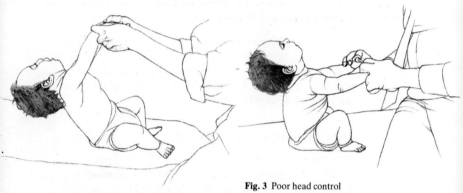

Fig. 2 Poor head control

Fig. 3 Poor head control

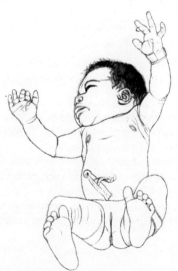

Fig. 4 Moro response

DEVELOPMENTAL SCREENING TESTS

6 weeks old

GROSS MOTOR

Head control (Pass by examination)

Method Pull the baby into a sitting position. This can be done by placing him supine, pulling gently on the hands or wrists, and then holding him in the sitting position.

Pass Hold his head upright and steady without wobbling (Fig. 1).

Note A newborn baby may not be able to hold his head steady, but head control is usually achieved by 6 weeks.

    If he cannot do this, it may indicate hypotonia, a cerebral disorder, or other factors such as sedation by drugs or an intercurrent illness (Figs 2 and 3).

Moro response (Pass by examination)

Method There are several methods of producing this response; for example: Support the head and shoulders on examiner's hands at about 15 cm from the table and suddenly allow the baby's head to drop back slightly.

OR

Use Moro's original method in which vibration is induced by suddenly slapping the bed.

Pass The response (extension of the arms followed by adduction towards the chest) is brisk and symmetrical (Fig. 4).

Note If the response is poor or asymmetrical, note which arm does not move properly. Failure could be due to weakness, fracture, dislocation or osteomyelitis. Ill babies often have a poor but symmetrical response.

    This response should disappear by 6 months. If it persists this may indicate a cerebral disorder, particularly if it reappears after having disappeared.

    Persistence of other primitive reflexes, especially asymmetrical tonic neck reflex, has the same significance.

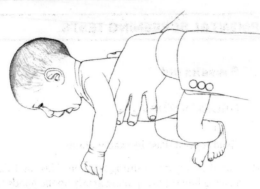

Fig. 5 Ventral suspension

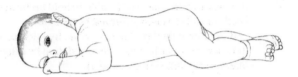

Fig. 6 Prone position

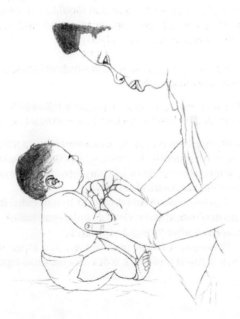

Fig. 7 Stares

Ventral suspension (Pass by examination)

Method   Hold the baby in ventral suspension.

Pass   The head is in line with or higher than the body, and the hips are semi-extended (Fig. 5).

Note   If he cannot do this, then it has the same significance as lack of head control. During the examination it is possible to elicit Galant's response: scratch gently, with a finger or pin, the skin of the infant's back, from the shoulder downwards, about 3 cm lateral to the spine. The baby's bottom will swing to the stimulated side. This is a very consistent response which is present at term and should disappear by 10 months. It is clearly absent when the muscles are weak, but has no other use.

Prone position (Pass by examination)

Method   Place the baby face down on a flat surface (Fig. 6).

Pass   He lifts his head, at least momentarily, and often as far as 45° from the surface. All babies can at least lift the head a little by 6 weeks.

Note   Failure to lift the head has the same significance as in 'Head control'.
Some babies who later have severe spasticity can lift their heads particularly well at this age (due to increased extensor tone).

FINE MOTOR AND VISION

Stares (Pass by examination or history)

Method   Look at the baby's face. Also ask mother: 'Does baby watch you while feeding?'

Pass   He stares at a face or his mother says he does (Fig. 7).

Note   No response may indicate poor vision or blindness, especially if associated with wandering eye movements.

Follows horizontally to 90° (Pass by examination)

Method   Put the child on his back with his face turned to one side. Hold a red woollen ball about 25 cm in front of the child's face. Gently shake it to attract his attention and then move it slowly from one side to the other, crossing his face.

Pass   The eyes alone, or the head and eyes together, cross the mid-line and travel through at least 90° in following the woollen ball (Fig. 8a–c).

Note   If the baby does not follow the ball the test should be repeated at least 3 times with a few minutes' interval between each testing. If he still does not follow the ball, he may have poor vision.

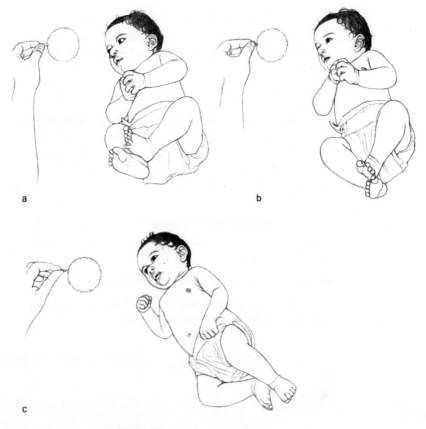

a   b

c

Fig. 8(a)–(c) Follows horizontally to 90°

HEARING AND SPEECH

Rattle or bell, 15 cm at ear level (Pass by examination)

Method   Hold the rattle or bell so that the child cannot see it. Sound it quietly for 3–5 s at 15 cm at ear level with 5 s pauses. Increase loudness if no response.

Pass   The baby quietens to this sound — the commonest response (Fig. 9). Also pass if he shows any other satisfactory response such as turning or widening of the eyes or if there is a change in breathing pattern.

Note   If the child does not respond, try again after a short while. If there is no response, repeat the test again after 2 weeks. Ask the parents if the baby can hear. If the parents do not think the child can hear, ask them to observe and to return in about 2 weeks' time.

Startle response (Pass by examination or history)

Method   Clap suddenly at ear level at 30 cm or ask parents if they think the child can hear, e.g. response to a sudden noise, such as the door being shut in another room or when the telephone rings.

Pass   He stiffens, blinks, screws up his eyes, extends his limbs or cries.

Note   If the child does not pass any of the above two tests he should be referred for paediatric audiological assessment.

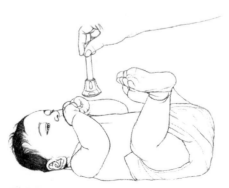

Fig. 9 Bell 15 cm away, at ear level (baby quietens)

SOCIAL BEHAVIOUR AND PLAY

Smiles (Pass by history or examination)

Method   Smile at the child. Do not stimulate by touch or sound. Ask parents if the child smiles.

Pass   The child smiles without any stimulation in response to examiner's or parent's face; also pass if parents say he smiles.

Note   If the baby does not pass, be suspicious. It may represent developmental delay, but should be assessed together with other tests. Spontaneous smiling may just begin at this age.
About 90% of babies have started to smile in response to an adult's smile by 6 weeks. At this age a baby may attempt to attract an adult's attention by smiling.

Turns to regard observer's face (Pass by history or examination)

Method   Put the child on his back. Bring your face within 30 cm (12 inches) of the child, and watch to see if he turns towards you. Ask the parents if the child turns to look at them.

Pass   The child looks at examiner, or parents say he does; also pass if he watches mother while feeding.

Note   Failure has the same significance as in 'Smiles'.

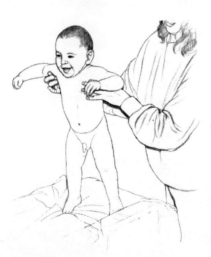

Fig. 10 Downward parachute response

6—8 months old

GROSS MOTOR

Bears weight on legs (Pass by examination)

Method   Hold the child upright in vertical suspension and rest his feet on a table or bed. Relax support but do not release.

Pass   Supports his weight on his legs.

Note   If he does not bear weight, this may represent weakness, hypotonia or hypertonia. Scissoring of legs (crossing the legs) will be unusual at this age, but if present may be due to spasticity. Floppy infants also fail — there are many causes of floppiness, including many benign causes.
   Failure also may be due to developmental delay, cerebral palsy or social deprivation.
   Check for muscle tone and also mobility of ankles, knees, hips and elbows. In hypotonia, excessive joint movement (hyperextensibility) is present and the limbs feel floppy. Children with hypotonia and hyperextensible joints do not bear weight but adopt a 'sitting on air' position. These children later shuffle or hitch on their bottom; they do not crawl. They walk late, at 23–30 months of age, and subsequently they will be normal in gross motor development and in intelligence, but mild inco-ordination due to mild hypotonia may persist.

Downward parachute response (Pass by examination)

(This is also known as the saving, propping or protective reaction.)

Method   Hold the child upright in vertical suspension, about 30 cm (1 foot) from a table or bed and rapidly lower him to land on the surface.

Pass   Lower limbs extend and abduct as the baby lands (Fig. 10).

Note   This response is present in some babies at 4 months and in almost all at 6 months.
   An asymmetrical parachute response may occur in weakness or spasticity of a limb and if a hip is dislocated. Fracture and infection of the limb should also be looked for. Failure also has the same significance as in 'Bears weight on legs'.

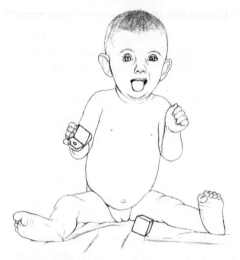

Fig. 11 Sits with support

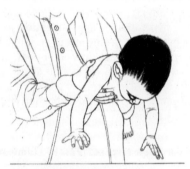

Fig. 12 Forward parachute response

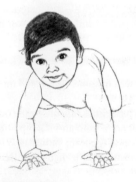

Fig. 13 Crawls

Sits with support (Pass by examination or history)

Method   Hold the child in a sitting position on a table or bed to see how well he can hold his head steady and whether his back is straight. Ask parents if baby can sit propped up, for instance by using a cushion.

Pass   Sits well with support or there is a positive history (Fig. 11).

Note   Failure may have the same significance as in 'Bears weight on legs'.

The balancing reactions may be tested during the examination by tilting the child to one side. At 4 months the child will tilt his head to 30° to keep his head upright and eyes level; at 5 months the spine curves to compensate.

Forward parachute response (Pass by examination)

Method   Hold the infant in prone suspension and suddenly tilt towards the examination couch.

Pass   Upper limbs and fingers abduct and extend (Fig. 12).

Note   This is another saving or propping or protective reaction, which is present by 9–12 months. If it is still not present at 12 months, it may represent developmental delay. These are not learned but inherited reactions.

Another such response which appears in the middle of the first year, is rolling. It may be tested by placing the child on his back on a hard surface and initiating rolling by gently pulling one of his legs. The child completes the roll and positions his arms by the sides of his chest. The parents will usually give a clear history of the child's ability to roll over from front to back which he will do first, and later from back to front. Most children can do this by 8–9 months.

Crawls (Pass by examination or history)

Method   See if the baby can crawl or ask parents if he crawls.

Pass   The child crawls or parents say he does (Fig. 13).

Note   The baby begins to crawl from 6 months; 90% of babies will crawl by 9 months. However, some babies do not crawl, but move about by shuffling on the buttocks or by rolling or creeping. These babies walk late (at 22–24 months); they are normal, but show a deviation of normal motor development. Thus, not crawling is not of major clinical significance, provided all other developmental milestones are normal.

FINE MOTOR AND VISION

Reaches out to grasp (palmar grasp) (Pass by examination or history)

Method   The child sits on a parent's lap so that he can easily reach out with his hands to a table. Place a brick, a small car or any other bright toy within easy reach and encourage him to pick it up.

Pass   The child picks up or tries to reach the toy. If he picks it up, note the grasp which is usually palmar, i.e. he uses the whole palm and fingers to hold the toy.

Note   If the baby does not reach out by 6 months, this indicates some developmental delay.

Transfer and mouths (Pass by examination or history)

Method   Give a brick to the child. Observe whether or not he passes it from one hand to the other and puts it in his mouth.

Pass   The child transfers (passes from one hand to the other) or mouths the brick (Fig. 14). If he does not transfer, encourage him by giving another brick. He may then transfer the first brick to the other hand in order to take the second one.

Note   The average age for passing this examination is about 6 months; by age 8 months 90% will do it.

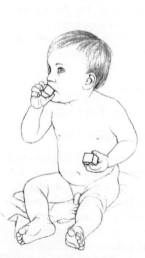

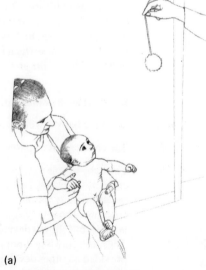

(a)

Fig. 14 Transfers and mouths   **Fig. 15(a)–(c)** Follows fallen toy

Fixes on small objects (Pass by examination)

Method   Drop a raisin or a Smartie on a table, which should be covered with a green cloth (if possible) to give good contrast. Smaller objects like 'silver balls' (0.3 mm in size) or 'hundreds and thousands' (cake decorations) may also be used.

Pass   Looks at the raisin or Smartie. If he fails to look, point to the object and attract his attention.

Note   Failure to fix his eyes on the object may represent visual inattention or poor eyesight. Repeat the test with a larger object such as a brick. If wandering movements or nystagmus are present, visual handicap is likely. It is important to arrange a detailed assessment of vision and an ocular examination.

Follows fallen toys (red woollen ball) (Pass by examination)

Method   The child sits on a parent's lap. Hold a bright toy or a red woollen ball in front of him. While he is looking at the object, drop it so that it falls. Do not move hand.

Pass   The child looks down to see the object (Fig. 15a–c). Test twice, if he does not look down.

Note   Failure to watch the falling toy object has the same significance as in 'Fixes on small objects'.

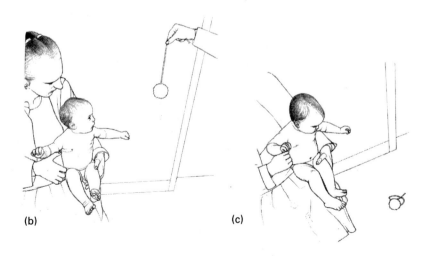

(b)   (c)

HEARING AND SPEECH

Vocalises (Pass by examination or history)

Method   Observe to see if the baby babbles and uses several syllables.

Pass   Babble and coos are heard; also pass if parents say they hear them.

Note   Vocalisation begins within the first month. At first, monosyllabic babbles such as cooing sounds ('ah', 'muh', 'goo', 'ba', 'da', 'ka') develop, and then polysyllables ('dad-dad', 'mum-mum', 'ga-ga'). At about 6 months, 50%; by 9 months, 90%. If there is no vocalisation, this may suggest a hearing deficit; it may be also due to an overall developmental delay.

Laughs (Pass by examination or history)

Method   Observe for loud laughs or high-pitched happy squeals.

Pass   The child laughs or parents say he does.

Note   If he has not started to laugh, this may have the same significance as in 'Vocalises'. Babies begin to laugh at about 2 months, certainly by 3 months all babies should laugh.

Responds to own name (Pass by examination or history)

Method   The child sits on a parent's lap. Stand beside and behind the child, making sure you are out of vision. Whisper the child's name several times from about 20 cm (1 foot) at ear level. Repeat twice more if the child does not respond. Ask parents if the baby can recognise his own name. Also ask parents if he can hear.

Pass   The baby turns to the direction of the voice; also pass if parents give a clear history that the baby will turn his head when his name is called softly.

Note   Response may be brisker on one side than the other. If he does not turn to localise sound or if there is no history of a response, this may indicate deafness or be a part of global delay as in 'Vocalises'.

Distraction hearing test (Pass by examination)

Performed at ear level at 1 m (3 feet) distance; cup and spoon, rattle, voice — 'ss-ss', 'oo-oo' and name — are used. The rattle is held at 30 cm (1 foot). Two persons are required for this test: one observer and one tester.

Method   The child is placed squarely on the parent's lap, facing one of a pair of observers. His attention is held by the observer moving an attractive soundless toy just out of reach. All the adults must keep quiet; it is important to point this out to the parents. The observer holding the toy suddenly hides it behind her back or keeps it still. At that moment, the other tester makes the sound which is being used as a stimulus at ear level. It is essential that this should be done slightly behind the child and out of vision. Both ears must be tested. All the stimuli should be used at about 40 dB in loudness.

(a) Rattle: those usually used are the Manchester and Nuffield rattles. They must be used very softly at about 30 cm (1 foot) from the baby's ear.

(b) Cup and spoon: use a china cup and a metal teaspoon. The spoon is run gently round the rim of the cup at 1 m (3 feet) from the baby's ear. Do not rattle the spoon in the cup.

(c) Voice at 1 m (3 feet): (i) a high-pitched sound, usually 'ss-ss', (ii) a low-pitched sound, such as 'oo-oo', (iii) a little conversation, always including the baby's name, such as 'Mary, can you hear me?' or 'Look here John'.

(a)   (b)

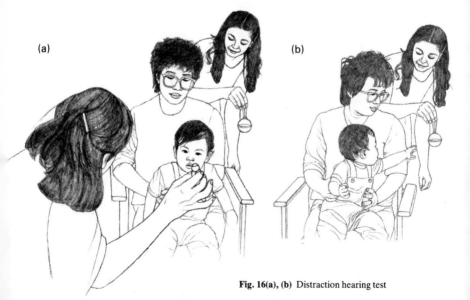

Fig. 16(a), (b) Distraction hearing test

The room must be quiet. The ambient sound level (background noise) should not be more than 30 dB, but this is difficult to achieve. The sound stimuli should be used initially at 40 dB. In order to use the sound correctly, it is important to obtain a sound-level meter to become accustomed to using the stimulus softly enough. A sound-level meter can usually be found at a referral centre. All examiners doing a hearing test must have used a meter at least once, and they should have their own hearing tested if there is any doubt about it.

Pass   The child instantly turns his head towards the sound in all the test items performed (Fig. 16a, b).

Note   If failed, the test may have to be repeated because it could be a temporary failure due to otitis media or wax. Check ears.

Partial deafness, especially high-tone loss, may be missed by this method. Some children are slow to respond, and one ear may be sharper than the other. If the hearing test is failed, a full audiological assessment should be done without delay.

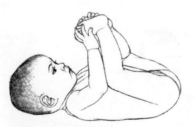

Fig. 17 Hand and foot regard

SOCIAL BEHAVIOUR AND PLAY

Puts everything to mouth (Pass by examination or history)

Method   Observe whether the child puts bricks or toys into his mouth.

Pass   The child puts objects into his mouth; also pass if parents say he does.

Note   Almost all children should be doing this by 8 months.

Hand and foot regard (Pass by examination or history)

Method   Ask parents whether the child plays with his hands and feet and tries to put a foot in his mouth.

Pass   Parents give a positive history or you observe the child with a foot in the mouth (Fig. 17).

Note   This starts at about 4 months and should disappear by 9 months. Persistence beyond 1 year may indicate developmental delay.
   Failure of regard at a younger age may also indicate developmental delay.

Plays peek-a-boo (Pass by examination or history)

Method   Make a 1 cm hole in the middle of an A4 size sheet of paper. Hide your face behind the paper and peep through the hole. Then look around the paper on the same side twice and each time say 'peek-a-boo'. Look through the hole to see if the child looks at the place where the face appeared.

Pass   The child looks in the direction of where the face appeared.

Note   If the child is unable to play peek-a-boo, it may be due to developmental delay or poor vision.

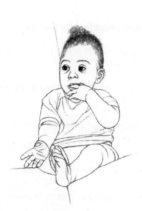

Fig. 18(a) Gets to sitting position

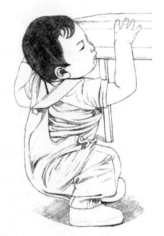

Fig. 18(b) Pulls to standing position

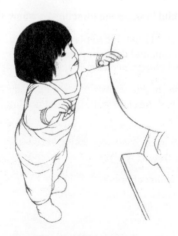

Fig. 19 Walks holding furniture

1 year old

GROSS MOTOR

Gets to sitting position (Pass by examination or history)

Method Lay the child on his back and watch what he can do. Ask parents if the child can rise to a sitting position from lying down: 'Will baby sit up himself from lying position?'

Pass The child is observed sitting up or parents say he does (Fig. 18a).

Note If he cannot sit up by himself, this may be due to developmental delay or cerebral palsy.

'Floppy infants' also do not pass — there are many causes of floppiness, including some benign causes. Some only have congenital joint laxity, some have a neuromuscular disorder and others a simple muscular hypotonia which improves with age, producing a normal child. These babies are somewhat unsteady and are rather late in walking.

Pulls to standing position (Pass by examination or history)

Method Put the child into a sitting position near a chair and watch to see if he can get to the standing position. Ask parents if the child can pull himself to standing without help from a person or while holding onto a solid object such as a chair.

Pass The child is observed pulling himself to standing or parents say he does (Fig. 18b).

Note If the child cannot stand, it has the same significance as in 'Gets to sitting position'.

Walks holding furniture (Pass by examination or history)

Method Put the child by a chair to see if he walks alongside it. Ask parents if the child walks around holding their hand or furniture.

Pass The child is observed walking holding the furniture or parents say he does (Fig. 19).

Note If the child cannot do this, it may have the same significance as in 'Gets to sitting position'.

Walks alone (Pass by examination or history)

Method   Observe the child as he walks.

Pass   The child walks well with good balance and without too many falls; also pass if parents say he can walk.

Note   If he cannot walk at this age, he is still probably normal. The average age for walking is around 14 months.

Many children have an unusual walking habit during the second year, and if they get around by bottom shuffling they may be very mobile but walk late (22–24 months).

Watch out for tiptoeing which, if persistent, may be due to spasticity in the legs. It is usually accompanied by scissoring when the child is held in a vertical position.

FINE MOTOR AND VISION

Points with index finger (Pass by history)

Method   Ask parents if the child points with the index finger at objects he wishes to handle, or to happenings which interest him.

Pass   Parents say he does.

Note   If the child does not point, it may indicate developmental delay, or poor hand–eye co-ordination due to visual impairment, weakness or ataxia.

Also note preferred hand of use. Constant fisting or hesitation to use one hand consistently may be indicative of hemiplegia or some other weakness of that hand (this may be confirmed by the forward parachute response, when abnormal posturing may be noted).

Casts (Pass by examination or history)

Method   Give the child a toy and see if he throws it onto the floor. Ask parents if he deliberately drops or throws toys or bricks and watch them fall to the floor.

Pass   The child is seen to cast or parents say he does.

Note   This is a normal feature of children at 12–15 months and should disappear by 18 months. Persistence beyond 18 months or failure to do it by 15 months may be associated with developmental delay. Children with visual impairment also do not cast.

Pincer grasp (Pass by examination)

Method The child sits on a parent's lap so that he can easily reach out with his hands to a table. Place small objects such as Smarties (or raisins) or 'hundreds and thousands' (cake decorations) within easy reach. It is best to put one Smartie (or raisin) at a time on a green felt or towel. Encourage him to pick up. The observer may demonstrate or point to attract his attention.

Pass The child picks up the Smartie or raisin with neat pincer grasp — between thumb and tip of index finger (Fig. 20a–d).

Note If the child does not pick up the object it has the same significance as in 'Points with index finger'. Many children at this age will pick up or reach out for a smaller object such as 'hundreds and thousands' (1 mm). This is a good test for near vision at this age.

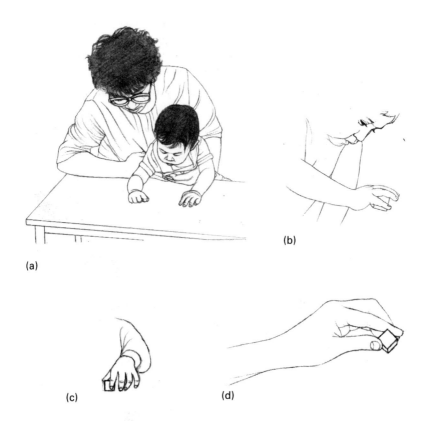

(a)

(b)

(c)

(d)

Fig. 20(a) Pincer grasp; (b) primitive (first-stage) grasp — whole hand approach; (c) intermediate (second-stage) grasp — with thumb and index finger use; (d) neat pincer grasp

Holds 2 bricks and bangs them together (Pass by examination)

Method   Give the child 2 bricks, one in each hand. Encourage him by showing him what to do with them. Do not touch the child's hands, but several imitations of the banging movement are allowed.

Pass   The child bangs the bricks (Fig. 21). It may take a few seconds for him to start doing it.

Note   If the child does not hold the bricks and play with them, it has the same significance as in 'Points with index finger'.

HEARING AND SPEECH

Turns to sound of name (Pass by examination or history)

Method   Seat the child on a parent's lap, facing one of a pair of examiners. The other examiner stands behind but to one side of the parents and out of vision. The child's name is called softly. Ask parent if the child knows and immediately turns in response to his own name.

Pass   The child turns his head definitely in response to his name; also pass if parents say he does.

Note   If he does not respond, there may be a hearing deficit; there may also be overall developmental delay. Children begin speech with babbling and cooing, and baby jargon appears later. Then he will turn to his own name. He will usually do this by 10 months. If in any doubt, carry out a full audiological assessment. See 'Distraction hearing test' (p.00).

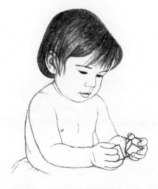

Fig. 21 Holds 2 bricks and bangs them together

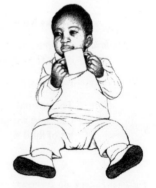

Fig. 22 Drinks from cup

Uses 'mama' and 'dada' (Pass by history)

Method   Ask parents if the child can say 'mama' and 'dada' and whether he uses them for the right person.

Pass   Parents say he uses these words appropriately. The child only rarely shows an examiner that he can correctly use these names, and they are not usually intelligible to outsiders.

Note   Words at this stage are a repetition of adult's playful sounds, such as 'mama', 'dada' and 'ta'. Some normal children do not use any words at this age.

Understands several words (Pass by history)

Method   Ask parents if he understands words such as cup, ball, car and the names of his brothers and sisters.

Pass   Parents say he understands.

Note   If does not understand anything, check hearing.

Distraction hearing test (Pass by examination)

This test only needs to be done if child was not tested at 8 months, or if there is doubt, or if he does not turn in response to his name.

Method   As on page 27.

Pass   As on page 27.

Note   Habituation (or boredom) occurs quickly at this age, so the test may be difficult to do.

SOCIAL BEHAVIOUR AND PLAY

Drinks from cup (Pass by history)

Method   Ask parents if the child can hold a cup without a spout and drink from it without spilling much.

Pass   Parents say he does (Fig. 22).

Note   The normal range for this continues well beyond 16 months. Children with poor hand–eye co-ordination or ataxia spill a lot of fluid while drinking.

Indicates wants (not by crying) (Pass by history)

Method   Ask parents how the child lets them know what he requires: 'How does your child let you know when he wants something, such as a toy or a drink?'

Pass   The child indicates by pointing, pulling or asking for the object by its correct name.

Note   Do not pass if the child only cries to indicate what he wants. Inability to indicate what he wants is normal until at least 15 months.

Plays pat-a-cake (Pass by examination or history)

Method   Demonstrate hand-clapping a few times (parents may also demonstrate it) and ask the child to clap as well.

Pass   The child claps or parents say he does (Fig. 23).

Note   This is simple hand-clapping. Only a few children may participate in actually playing 'pat-a-cake', which is rhythmic clapping in tune with the parents or the examiner. If he does not clap by 14 months, it may indicate developmental delay.

Waves good-bye (Pass by history or examination)

Method   Ask parents if he can wave good-bye by waving at himself or them when he leaves the room.

Pass   Parents say he does or he demonstrates it (Fig. 24).

Note   If he will not wave, he may just be shy. The normal age range goes up to at least 15 months.

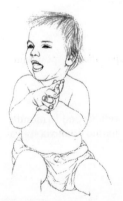

Fig. 23 Plays pat-a-cake (simple clapping)

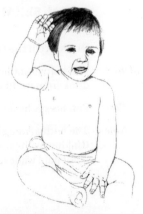

Fig. 24 Waves good-bye

18 months old

GROSS MOTOR

Walks backwards (Pass by examination or history)

Method   Ask the child to walk backwards (demonstrate if necessary) or ask parents if he can do this.

Pass   The child walks at least two steps backwards or parents say he does.

Note   This test is possible only if the child can already walk and run independently. The normal range for walking continues up to 18 months, or even later in those with a different method of getting around, such as bottom shuffling or creeping.

Great difficulty, or lateness, in walking, may be due to developmental delay or cerebral palsy. A normal child may not be able to walk backwards until he is nearly 2 years old, but the average child does it at 15 months.

Carries toys while walking (Pass by examination or history)

Method   Observe or ask parents if the child can carry a large toy such as a teddy-bear or car while walking.

Pass   The child carries a large toy or parents say he does (Fig. 25).

Note   Inability to do this has the same significance as in 'Walks backwards'.

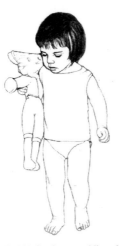

Fig. 25 Carries toys while walking

Climbs stairs (Pass by history)

Method   Ask parents if the child ascends stairs unaided. He may use rail for support, but not by holding onto a person or crawling.

Pass   Parents say he does.

Note   If he is not able to do this, it has the same significance as in 'Walks backwards'. This test is clearly difficult to apply in those families who live on one level.

Climbs onto chair (Pass by history)

Method   Ask parents if the child can climb onto chairs.

Pass   Parents say he does (Fig. 26).

Note   If he cannot climb, it has the same significance as in 'Walks backwards'. Children with hypotonia or ataxia are unsteady and will hesitate to climb.

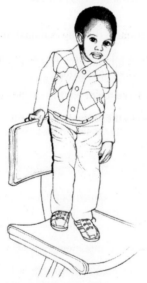

Fig. 26 Climbs onto a chair

FINE MOTOR AND VISION

Delicate pincer grasp (Pass by examination)

Method The child sits on a parent's lap so that he can easily reach out with his hands to a table. In front of him, on the table, place a small object like a Smartie or raisin; 'hundreds and thousands' may also be used. Encourage him to pick it up and watch how he does it.

Pass The child picks up by using thumb and index finger.

Note Do not pass if he uses any other finger; also fail if he misses it on several attempts or if his hand is shaky – this may be due to inco-ordination.

He may not pass the test if there is poor eye–hand co-ordination; and children with poor vision may also fail.

Watch for nystagmus, squint or wandering eye movements.

Children with intellectual impairment or cerebral palsy may perform this test later or may never do it.

Scribbles (with preferred hand) (Pass by examination or history)

Method Put a pencil in the child's hand and encourage him to scribble on a piece of paper. Parents may be asked to encourage him. Also ask parents whether he scribbles at home.

Pass Makes two or more purposeful markings on the paper. Do not pass if he stabs at the paper. Also pass if parents say he scribbles.

Note Inability to scribble has the same significance as in 'Delicate pincer grasp'.

Watch for very marked inco-ordination, as this might indicate a neurological problem.

Turns pages (Pass by examination or history)

Method Give the child a baby book and watch how he turns the pages or ask parents if he can turn pages.

Pass The child is seen to turn pages (two or more pages at a time are allowed). Observe whether he is interested. Also pass if parents say he does.

Note Inability to do this has the same significance as in 'Delicate pincer grasp'.

Builds tower of 3 or 4 bricks (Pass by examination)

Method   The child sits on a parent's lap so that he can easily reach out with his hands to a table. Place 4 bricks on the table in front of the child, and encourage him to build a tower. Tester or parents may demonstrate, and one brick at a time may be handed to the child.

Pass   Makes a tower with at least 3 bricks, so that it does not fall — three attempts are allowed (Fig. 27).

Note   The age at which children are able to build towers of 3–4 bricks goes up to at least 2 years. The average age is about 18 months.

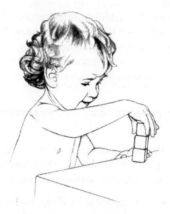

Fig. 27 Builds tower with 3 bricks

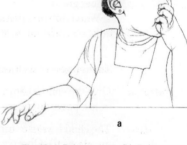

a

Fig. 28(a) Points to nose; (b) Points to ear

b

HEARING AND SPEECH

Jabbers continually (Pass by history and examination)

Method Ask parents if he jabbers loudly and continually to himself while playing (a dictionary defines jabbering as speaking volubly and with little sense, or uttering words rapidly and indistinctly).

Pass Parents say he does and if observed.

Note If he does not jabber, it may be normal but could be due to defective hearing, mental retardation, deprivation, a developmental speech disorder (developmental dysphasia) or a psychiatric disorder such as infantile autism.

Some children have delayed auditory maturation. As a distraction hearing test is difficult at this age, if poor hearing is suspected early referral to an audiologist is necessary.

Utters 3 or more words other than 'mama' and 'dada' (Pass by history)

Method Ask parents how many recognisable single words with meaning the child can use.

Pass Parents say 3 or more words, apart from 'mama' and 'dada'.

Note Some normal children use only an occasional words at this stage and this may be due to developmental dysphasia. There are still at least 3% of children who do not say 3 words by 18 months.

Check the family history, because developmental dysphasia may be inherited; it is also common in boys, and in those with left-handedess or ambidexterity. Later, these children may have mild reading and writing problems.

If there is no speech, it may have the same significance as in 'Jabbers continually'.

Points to eyes, nose and mouth (Pass by examination or history)

Method Ask parents if the child can point to his eyes, nose and mouth, and ask them to demonstrate. They are allowed to ask the child to point to a doll's eyes, nose or mouth.

Pass Performs or parents say he does (Fig. 28a–b).

Note This test is for comprehension of speech but not for hearing, because loudness of voice is not taken into consideration.

At 18 months, 50% of normal children pass this test. Nearly 10% do not pass at 2 years. Inability to do the test may therefore be normal, but could indicate developmental delay or hearing loss, if the result of other tests are abnormal.

Obeys simple instruction: 'Close the door' (Pass by examination or history)

Method   Ask parents if child obeys simple instructions such as 'Close the door' or 'Put it back'. Also ask them to demonstrate.

Pass   The child performs or parents say he does.

Note   If the child does obey a simple instruction, this has the same significance as in 'Points to eye, nose and mouth'. However many children (over 10%) will not do this until 2½ years.

SOCIAL BEHAVIOUR AND PLAY

Holds spoon: gets food to mouth (Pass by history)

Method   Ask parents if the child holds spoon and gets food safely to his mouth without too much mess.

Pass   Parents say he does (Fig. 29).

Note   10% of children cannot do this by 24 months. When a child is unable to use a spoon by 2½ years, consider mental retardation, emotional disturbance or deprivation.

Children with inco-ordination also use a spoon poorly and they spill food.

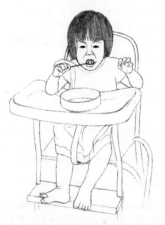

Fig. 29 Holds spoon — gets food to mouth

Explores environment (Pass by history)

Method   Ask parents if the child explores the environment by vigorous activities (indoor and outdoor) — running, climbing, jumping and opening doors — 'Goes into everything'.

Pass   Parents say he does.

Note   If he does not show interest in his surroundings it may have the same significance as in 'Holds spoon: gets food to mouth'.

Takes off shoes and socks (Pass by history)

Method   Ask parents if the child can take off his shoes and socks.

Pass   Parents say he does.

Note   If he is unable to do this, it may have the same significance as in 'Holds spoon: gets food to mouth'.

Indicates toilet needs (Pass by history)

Method   Ask parents how the child indicates toilet needs — what he does when he likes to go to toilet or how he indicates when wet or soiled.

Pass   Parents say that he indicates by any means: pointing, showing potty or toilet; a few children may say 'poo' or another word.

Note   Some parents have a programme of training for bowel and bladder control, whereas others have a very liberal and relaxed approach. Therefore, this stage of development depends to some extent on the parents' attitude as well as the child's mental and physical ability.

2–2½ years old

GROSS MOTOR

Climbs and descends stairs (Pass by history)

Method   Ask parents how the child gets up stairs.

Pass   Walks up and down the stairs, holding rail or wall, but not a person. Two feet to a step is allowed but crawling is not.

Note   If the child is unable to go up and down stairs, it may be due to developmental delay or cerebral palsy.

By 22 months, 90% of children can walk up stairs.

Children with inco-ordination and ataxia are hesitant to use stairs.

Jumps in place (Pass by examination or history)

Method   Ask the child to jump from a standing position across the width of a sheet of A4 size paper (20 cm). Parents or tester may demonstrate how to do this.

Pass   The child raises both feet off the floor at the same time and jumps across. He is not allowed to run before he jumps or hold anything for support. Do not count a pass if he hops.

Note   If the child is unable to do this, it may have the same significance as in 'Climbs and descends stairs'.

Many 2-year-old children cannot jump, and 10% of children still lack this skill by their third birthday.

Kicks ball (Pass by examination or history)

Method   Place a ball (like a tennis ball) in front of the child. Ask him to kick it. Demonstrate once, if required. Ask parents if he can kick a ball forwards.

Pass   The child kicks the ball forward without holding any support; also pass if parents say he does (Fig. 30).

Note   If the child cannot kick, it has the same significance as in 'Climbs and descends stairs'.

FINE MOTOR AND VISION

Picks up 'hundreds and thousands' (Pass by examination)

Method Sit the child comfortably on a parent's lap or on a small chair. Place one 'hundreds and thousands' (cake decorations) on a green felt or towel (or on the tester's palm) in front of him within easy reach. Ask him to pick it up. If he refuses, you can put several in front of him. Care should be taken that the child does not get any other clues as to the presence of the object. The tester may also point to the object.

Pass The child picks it up accurately and quickly.

Note 'Hundreds and thousands' are about 1 mm in diameter. If the child is unable to pick one up because he could not see it then careful ophthamological assessment is required.

If squint or nystagmus is seen, this may be significant. Referral to an ophthalmologist should then be prompt.

If the child does not pick it up accurately, or if his hands are shaky, it may be due to clumsiness or ataxia; children with cerebral palsy may also perform this test crudely.

This is a good test of near vision, but no data are available to indicate the age when inability to see tiny objects is abnormal. We suggest 2 years is abnormal, but the child's eyes should be carefully examined if he cannot do it at 15–18 months.

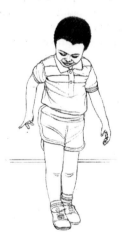

Fig. 30 Kicks ball

Imitates vertical line (Pass by examination and history)

Method　The child sits comfortably on a parent's lap or in his own chair, so that he is at comfortable writing level. Place a paper in front of him and draw 1–2 vertical lines about 5 cm long to demonstrate how to draw vertical lines. Give him a pencil and ask him to copy it: 'Draw a line the same as this one'.

Pass　The child draws one or more lines at least 2 cm long and not varying from the vertical line by more than 30° (Fig. 31). Lines do not have to be perfectly straight.

Note　If he cannot draw the line, it may indicate poor vision or developmental delay. A 2-year-old child would often be unable to draw the line and 10% of children cannot do this by their third birthday.

Build towers of 8 bricks (Pass by examination)

Method　The child sits comfortably on a parent's lap or on his own chair. Demonstrate once how to build a tower and ask him to build it. Give him one brick at a time.

Pass　The child builds a tower with 8 bricks (Fig. 32). He may have 3 attempts.

Note　Ten per cent of children still cannot do this correctly by 3½ years.

　　Watch for clumsiness and ataxia, signs of poor vision, or general evidence of developmental delay.

　　If he is unable to build, it may have the same significance as in 'Picks up "hundreds and thousands"'. Poor hand–eye co-ordination may be due to clumsiness or ataxia.

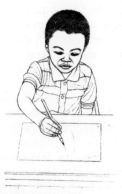

Fig. 31 Imitates vertical line

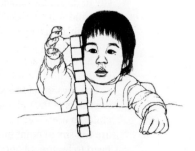

Fig. 32 Builds tower of 8 bricks

HEARING AND SPEECH

Uses plurals (Pass by examination or history)

Method Ask parents if the child uses plurals. As a test, place 3 bricks in front of the child and ask him: 'What are these?'

Pass Parents say he uses plurals or, when tested, the child answers using plurals, such as 'bricks's'.

Note Ninety per cent of children use plurals by their third birthday. If a child does not speak, remember to test his hearing.

Gives name (Pass by examination or history)

Method Ask the child: 'What is your name?' (parents are allowed to repeat the question for him). If only the first name is given, encourage him to give his last name. Parents may be asked if he can give his full name.

Note Ten per cent of children are still unable to give their first and last name by 3½ years. Test the hearing of these children. Always consider speech therapy in any child with delayed speech development.

Speech discrimination test (Pass by examination)

There are several methods for testing the hearing of children older than 2½ years. The commonest ones are the McCormick and Kendall Toy Tests.

Method The child sits on a small chair with a table in front of him, or on a parent's lap at a higher table. The examiner sits 1 m from the child on the other side of the table and brings out a box of 12 toys. Each of the toys is taken out of the box one by one and placed on the table (Fig. 33). As this is done the child is asked to give the name of each object. If he cannot or is too shy to do so, the examiner gives the name clearly. Sometimes the child will give an inappropriate name, e.g. 'sheep' instead of 'lamb' or 'gee-gee' for 'horse'. Then the examiner must give the right name for the test.

The toys in each test are listed below. They are in pairs or groups, with a view to testing discrimination of consonants.

The toys should be spread out in front of the child and members of the pairs should be well separated. When children are asked to show an examiner the toy, they often are too shy to point but will look at the object. The toys will need to be spread out to allow this 'pointing' with the eyes.

The examiner must have tested his voice against a sound-level meter. It is best for him to have the meter on his desk at the same distance as he is from the child. Often it is possible to determine the softest voice to which the child responds.

It is important to cover the mouth (usually with the lid of the toy-box, or with a hand) to prevent the child from lip-reading.

At the start of the test the examiner must name one or two toys, using normal speech to be certain that the child understands what to do. He should quieten his voice so that it produces 40 dB at the child's ears. Each of the toys must be named, and it is important not to look at them but at the child. In this way, it is possible to be certain that the child has heard correctly and has not been given visual clues. Some younger children will do the test successfully if they are asked to give the toys to the parent.

If the child picks up a toy, it must be replaced on the table before testing with another toy.

If the child does not become bored, it may be possible to test each ear independently by naming the toy from each side of the sound-level meter.

At the end of the test, the children often enjoy helping by putting the toys away in the box.

Toys in the matching groups used are:
plane/plate/gate
duck/cup
spoon/shoes
cow/house/mouse
fish/brick

Children with normal hearing can usually discriminate between all the toys at the minimal level of 35–40 dB(A).

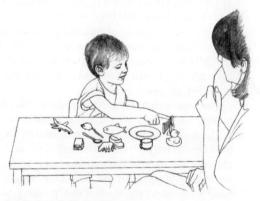

Fig. 33 Speech discrimination test

SOCIAL BEHAVIOUR AND PLAY

Plays alone (Pass by history)

Method   Ask parents if the child plays alone, quietly and contentedly near other children but not with them. This often includes role-play, such as combing a doll's hair.

Pass   Parents say he does and he plays with his friends (Fig. 34).

Note   There is a wide range in the ages at which children start to play with toys constantly. Some hyperactive children find it very difficult to concentrate by themselves.

Eats with spoon and fork (Pass by history)

Method   Ask parents if the child can feed himself using spoon and fork, without much spillage.

Pass   Parents say he does.

Note   This ability occurs late in children with inco-ordination and in those with mental handicap or other causes of developmental delay.

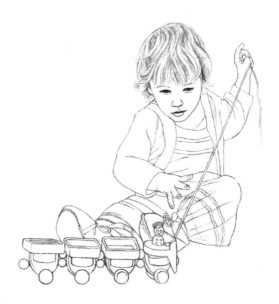

Fig. 34 Plays alone

Puts on clothes (Pass by history)

Method   Ask parents if the child can put on some clothes, such as shoes. He is not expected to button coats.

Pass   Parents say he can.

Note   There are about 10% of children who still cannot do this at 3 years.

Dry throughout day (Pass by history)

Method   Ask parents if the child is usually dry.

Pass   Parents say he is dry throughout the day. Also if he wets occasionally, but is normally dry throughout the day.

Note   It is unusual for a child not to have bladder control after 3 years. If there is persistent wetting (not an occasional accident), it is important to be certain that the urine is normal.

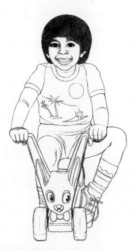

Fig. 35 Pedals tricycle

3 years old

GROSS MOTOR

Runs fast (Pass by history)

Method   Ask parents if the child can run fast without falling.

Pass   Parents say he does.

Climbs stairs in adult manner (Pass by history)

Method   Ask parents if the child walks alone upstairs with alternating feet, one on each step. The child may hold on to a banister rail.

Pass   Parents say he does; he may descend the stairs two feet to a step.

Pedals tricycle (Pass by history)

Method   Ask parents if the child can pedal a tricycle.

Pass   Parents say he is able to pedal forward 3 m (10 feet) or more on level ground (Fig. 35). Pedalling the tricycle downhill does not count as a pass, nor does propelling the tricycle by pushing the feet on the ground.

Note   If the child has had no opportunity to ride a tricycle, omit this question. Most children ride a tricycle by 2½ years.

It is very significant if a child who was able to ride a tricycle now finds it difficult; this suggests that the muscles are getting weak (as in muscular dystrophy).

Only 10% of children cannot use a tricycle by 3 years.

Stands on one foot for one second (Pass by examination)

Method   Demonstrate to the child how to stand on one foot (parents may also demonstrate). Ask the child to stand on one foot without holding on. Three attempts are allowed. Ask the child to stand on one leg, then the other, and then the first again.

Pass   The child stands on one foot for one second or more in 2 or 3 trials (Fig. 36).

Note   Ten per cent of children are unable to do this at 3½ years. Children with ataxia or weakness would fail this test.

FINE MOTOR AND VISION

Copies circle (Pass by examination)

Method   The child sits comfortably on a parent's lap or in his own chair, with a table at the comfortable writing level. Place a paper and pencil in front of him and ask him to copy the circle. Have a circle ready — roughly 3 cm (1 inch) radius, or draw a circle without the child seeing what you are doing, because copying a circle is different from imitation when the circle is drawn in front of him. Place it in front of the child. Do not name it or show him how to draw it, but say: 'Draw one like this' or 'Draw one like the picture'.

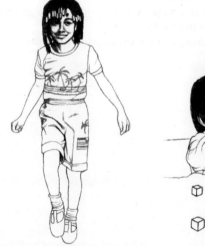

Fig. 36 Stands on one foot for 1 second

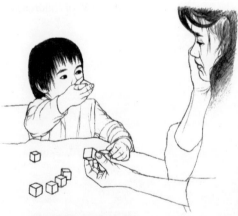

Fig. 37 Matches 2 colours

Pass The circle is drawn in any enclosed form — the end of the circle must be where it began. Circles not closed or made up of continuous round motions are not acceptable.

Note If the child cannot draw, repeat at 3½ years of age. About 20% of normal 3-year-old children may not draw a circle. However, if unable to do so at 4 years, the child may have poor hand–eye co-ordination or perceptual difficulties. Check his vision carefully and consider referral for developmental assessment.

Threads beads well (Pass by examination

Method Ask the child to thread 2 beads on a stick or on a thread.

Pass The child threads the beads well.

Note Observe how the child was threading. He should not have a tremor (shaking). Tremor may indicate inco-ordination. Children with poor vision will have difficulty in threading.

Matches 2 colours (Pass by examination)

Method Place 8 bricks — 2 each of the four primary colours (red, green, yellow, blue) — in front of the child on the table. Select the red one and ask him what colour it is. If he is unable to name the colour (which is the usual response), ask him to select one of the same colour: 'Give me another brick same colour as this' (Fig. 37). Put both back on the table. Repeat with yellow next and then test blue and green similarly. Do not tell him if the choices are correct.

Pass The child identifies correctly 2 of the 4 colours (he will identify red and yellow correctly, but may confuse blue and green).

Note If the test is failed, it may have the same significance as in 'Copies circle'; however, children with colour blindness may fail all colours (see pp. 75–77).
   Colour recognition is possible by 3½–4 years; the child will pick the correct brick by colour when asked 'Show me the red brick', but may not name it until 4½–5 years.

HEARING AND SPEECH

Uses prepositions (Pass by history)

Method Ask parents if the child uses prepositions. (Preposition: word marking the relation between the noun or pronoun it governs and another word, e.g. 'Put the cup *on* the table'.) This can be tested by giving the child a brick and asking him to put it *on* the table, and *behind, in front of* and *under* the chair.

Pass Parents say he does or the child is observed using them (for 3 out of 4 prepositions).

Note If failed, the test may have the same significance as under 'Jabbers continually' (see p. 4).

Ten per cent of children do not use prepositions until after 4½ years. Failure to use intelligible speech by 4 years is significant; full assessment, including hearing, is then required.

Uses sentences of 4 words (Pass by examination or history)

Method Ask parents if the child uses small sentences using at least 4 words (check, if possible, by sustained conversation).

Pass Parents say he does or he is heard to use sentences.

Note Failure has the same significance as in 'Uses prepositions'.

Inability to make sentences is another indication of speech delay. Assessment by a speech therapist and testing of hearing is advisable if a child cannot do this by 3½ years.

Gives full name, sex and age (Pass by examination or history)

Method Ask the child: 'What is your name?'; then: 'Are you a boy or a girl?'; and 'How old are you?' Parents may repeat the question. If the child gives only his first name, ask him to give his second (last name). The examiner may ask, for example, 'John who?'

Pass Gives understandable (not necessarily perfect) answers.

Note Under-stimulated children may not be able to give address correctly. Check with parents that the child has been told his address.

Ten per cent of children cannot give their full names by 3 years 9 months. Failure to do this by 4 years indicates delay.

SOCIAL BEHAVIOUR AND PLAY

Eats with knife and fork (Pass by history)

Method Ask parents if the child uses knife and fork for eating.

Pass Parents say he does.

Note If he does not use them, it has the same significance as in 'Holds spoon: gets food to mouth' (see p.42).

Goes to toilet alone (Pass by history)

Method Ask parents if the child goes to the toilet alone.

Pass Parents say he does.

Note Children with developmental delay frequently need adult help when they use the lavatory for defaecation.

Dresses with supervision (Pass by history)

Method Ask parents if the child can dress himself without help and inquire what help is needed.

Pass Parents say he puts on his clothes, knows the front from the back and they do not help him to dress.

Note The ability to dress is delayed in children with poor co-ordination and in those with developmental delay such as mental handicap.
Fifty per cent of children can do this by 3 years; 90% by about 3½ years.

Washes and dries hands (Pass by examination or history)

Method Ask parents if the child washes and dries his hands by himself.

Pass Parents say he does. Pass only if he can wash and dry all parts of hands without help, except for turning on taps that are out of reach. If necessary, check. Hands should be dry and completely free of soap.

Note If he cannot do it, it has the same significance as in 'Goes to toilet alone' (above).
The majority of children can do this by their second birthday and 90% just after their third birthday.

Separates from mother easily (Pass by history)

Method   Ask parents if the child can be left with a babysitter without becoming too upset.

Pass   Parents say he can separate from them relatively easily.

Note   Some children are never separated from their parents for several years and this must be taken into account when making an assessment.

4 years old

GROSS MOTOR

Hops on one foot for 2 metres forward (Pass by examination)

Method   Ask the child to hop on one (preferred) foot — do not let him hold on to anything. Parents or tester may demonstrate how to do it.

Pass   The child hops on one foot for about 2 m forward. The distance is not important, but the child should hop at least twice in a row.

Note   If he cannot do this, it may be due to weakness, clumsiness or ataxia. A careful neurological examination may identify the problem.
Children with hyperextensible joints may also have difficulty in hopping.

Climbs ladder/tree/slide (Pass by history)

Method   Ask parents if the child can climb up a ladder, tree or slide.

Pass   Parents say he does.

Note   If he does not do this, he may simply be a normal unadventurous child.

Stands on one foot for 5 seconds (Pass by examination)

Method   Ask the child to stand on one (preferred) foot without holding on. Time him using a watch. The child should be given 3 trials. Parents or tester may demonstrate how to do it

Pass   The child stands on one foot for 5 s or more in 2 out of 3 trials.

Note   If he refuses to do it, this bears the same significance as in 'Hops on one foot'.
The 50% centile is at 4½ years; 10% of children still do not do it by 5½ years.

Walks heel-to-toe (Pass by examination)

Method Show the child about 8 steps of heel-to-toe walking (tester should walk with the heel of one foot in front of and touching the toe of the other). Ask the child to walk similarly. He must be given 3 trials. (Parents or tester may compare this to a tightrope: '. . . as in the circus.' Parents or tester may demonstrate again if required.)

Pass The child walks in a straight line for 4 or more steps, placing his heel 2 cm (1 inch) or less in front of his toe, in 2 out of 3 trials (Fig. 38).

Note The mean age for this is 3 years 9 months and only 10% do not do it by 4 years 9 months.

   If failed, this test has the same significance as in 'Hops on one foot for 2 metres forward'.

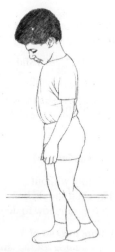

Fig. 38 Walks heel-to-toe

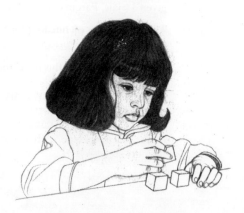

Fig. 39 Imitates bridge of 3 bricks

FINE MOTOR AND VISION

Copies cross and square (Pass by examination)

Method   As for 'Copies circle' (see p.52). Draw a circle and a cross about the same size, and ask the child to copy each separately. Tell him: 'Draw one like the picture', and point to each of them. If he is able to copy both correctly, then show him a square; do not demonstrate how to draw the square, and do not name it.

Pass   Draws a circle in any enclosed form and the two lines of the cross intersect at any point. The lines do not need to be straight or at right angles. The result of the square should have four approximate right angles at the corners. They should not be deformed with points or rounded corners.

Note   If he is not able to copy these designs, it has the same significance as in 'Copies circle'.

 Ninety per cent of children can copy a cross by 4 years 8 months. The square is more difficult; the 50th centile is at 4 years 7 months and the 90th centile at 6 years 3 months.

 At 4 years, the child may be unable to copy a square, but can only imitate it, i.e. draw it after demonstration.

 Demonstrate as follows: draw two sides first and then the other two opposite sides rather than drawing the square with a continuous motion (it may appear to be round to the child).

Imitates bridge of 3 bricks (Pass by examination)

Method   Tell the child to watch carefully while the bridge is being built. Place 2 bricks side by side, with less than a brick's space between, and not touching. Place the third brick on top of these, so that it covers the space between them. Give 3 bricks to the child and ask him to build a bridge like the one demonstrated. The bridge should be left standing for the child to copy, but pointing to the opening is not permitted.

Pass   The child copies the bridge correctly (Fig. 39). Eighty per cent of children can do this by 2 years 9 months and 90% by 3 years 6 months. If the 2 bricks on the bottom of the bridge are touching, do not point this out, but ask the child: 'Is your bridge like my bridge?'. He is allowed to correct himself, but no hints are allowed.

Note   If he cannot construct a bridge, this has the same significance as in 'Copies circle' (see p.52). It may also be due to poor hand–eye co-ordination which is present in some clumsy children.

Draws man with 3 parts (Pass by examination)

Method Give the child paper and a pencil and ask him to: 'Draw a man' or 'Draw your daddy'. Do not help, prompt or tell him to add any other parts. Ask 'Have you finished?' If he says 'yes', evaluate the drawing (Fig. 40).

Pass The child draws a head with 2 other parts. Most children can draw 6 parts. One point is given for each pair (ears, eyes, arms and legs) and also for each part which is not a pair (head, neck, body, nose, mouth, etc). If only one part of a pair is drawn, it is not counted.

Note If the child is unable to draw a man with three parts, it may have the same significance as in 'Copies circle' (see p.52) and may also represent poor body image, which a few clumsy children may have.

This scoring is the Denver Developmental Screening scoring and not the Goodenough-Harris 'Draw-a-man' Test scoring (see p.65). About 50% of children can draw this by 3 years 8 months and 90% by 4 years 8 months.

HEARING AND SPEECH

Counts up to 10 (Pass by examination or history)

Method Ask the child to count as far as he can.

Pass The child counts up to 10 without a mistake.

Note If failed, this test may represent psychosocial deprivation or developmental delay. Compare performance in other tests to assess the significance.

If hearing is in doubt, referral to an audiologist is mandatory.

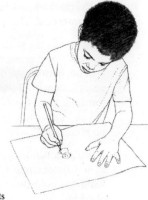

Fig. 40 Draws a man with 3 parts

Gives full name, age and address (Pass by examination or history)

Method Ask the child to say his name and then his age and address: 'What is your name?' If second name is not given, ask: '. . . who?' Ask for age and address separately: 'How old are you?', 'Where do you live?', 'What is your address?', etc. Parents may repeat the question, but no prompting is allowed.

Pass The child gives the details correctly. Check with parents to be certain it is correct.

Note Some children are very shy. However, psychosocial deprivation or developmental delay should be considered. If parents have not taught the child, he may not know his second name and address (especially if they have changed address recently).

At 2½ years, nearly 50% of children can give their first and second names; 90% by 3 years 5 months. Age and address are given at an older age.

If the child cannot give the information, this has the same significance as in 'Speaks fluently and clearly' (see p.67).

Recognises colours (Pass by examination or history)

Method Place red, blue, green and yellow bricks on a table (one of each colour) in front of the child. Ask him to point to or give the red brick, the blue brick and so on (if the child gives a brick, replace it on the table before the next colour is asked for). Do not indicate whether the answers are right or wrong. Do not ask him to name the colours. If he did not co-operate, ask parents if he can recognise colours, or repeat the test with parents requesting child.

Pass The child picks 3 of the 4 colours correctly or parents say he knows his colours.

Note Failure has the same significance as in 'Speaks fluently and clearly'. At 3 years, 50% can do this; at about 5 years, 90%.

SOCIAL BEHAVIOUR AND PLAY

Shares toys (Pass by history)

Method Ask parents if the child shares his toys with other children when they are playing.

Pass Parents say he shares and plays games co-operatively with other children.

Note If he does not share toys, ask what he plays with and if he mixes well. On its own, reluctance to share is of no significance, but if other behaviour is also abnormal, referral to child guidance may be necessary. It could be a manifestation of infantile autism or autistic behaviour in children with mental subnormality.

Brushes teeth (Pass by history)

Method Ask parents if the child brushes teeth himself.

Pass Parents say he does.

Note Examine to exclude any gum and teeth problems which may cause pain if his teeth are brushed.
　　　Some children do not brush their teeth because they have not been taught.

Dresses without supervision (Pass by history)

Method Ask parents if the child can dress himself or herself without supervision and can button (for boys, laces and ties are excluded; for girls, back buttons are excluded). Buttons need not be in the correct holes.

Pass Parents say the child does dress himself, including buttoning.

Note Fifty per cent can do this at 4 years, but the 90th centile is 5½ years.
　　　If unable to do this, it has the same significance as in 'Brushes teeth'.
　　　Intention tremor in children with ataxia and athetoid or choreiform movements may interfere with buttoning — if failed, full neurological assessment is required.

5 years old

GROSS MOTOR

Walks downstairs one foot per step (Pass by history)

Method Ask if the child can walk downstairs one foot per step.

Pass Parents say he can.

Note If the child cannot do this, it has the same significance as in 'Hops on one foot for 2 metres forward' (see p.57).

Bounces and catches ball (Pass by history or examination)

Method Ask the child to catch a tennis ball when it has bounced once. Parents (or tester) stand about 1 metre (3 feet) from the child and bounce the ball to him. The ball should bounce once halfway between tester and child and should reach him between the neck and waist. The child is allowed 3 attempts.

Pass The child catches the ball with hand or hands in 2 out of 3 attempts. He may catch the ball against his body using hands but not arms (if arms are used to catch the ball against his body, it would not be a pass).

Note By 2½ years most children can throw a ball overhand; 50% of children can catch a ball by 5 years and 90% by 6 years 3 months.

Walks backwards heel-to-toe (Pass by examination)

Method Demonstrate walking heel-to-toe backwards (walk placing the toe of one foot to the back of and touching the heel of the other). Ask the child to walk backwards similarly. He is asked to do this 3 times.

Pass Walks backwards in a straight line for 4 or more steps, placing his toe (2 cm) (1 inch) or less to back of other heel in 2 out of 3 trials.

Note Fifty per cent of children do this by 4 years 1 month and 90% by 5 years 7 months.

FINE MOTOR AND VISION

Copies triangle (Pass by examination)

Method The child sits comfortably on a chair so that he is at a comfortable writing level. Place a paper and pencil in front of him and ask him to copy the triangle. Have a triangle ready, size roughly 3 cm (1 inch) base length, or draw a triangle and place it in front of the child. Do not name it or show him how to draw it. Say 'Draw one like this' or 'Draw one like the picture'.

Pass The triangle is completed and the lines at the three corners touch each other. The corners must not be rounded.

Note If the child does not pass, test to see if he can copy a square (see p.59). Many children are only able to copy a triangle by 5½–6 years.

   If at 6 years he is unable to copy a square, then psychological assessment should be considered. This will detect mental subnormality or a specific problem if present.

Draws man with all features (Pass by examination)

Method   Give the child a pencil and eraser and ask him to draw a man on the blank paper. No encouragement or additional suggestion should be given.

Pass   The child draws all features correctly (a man with more than 6 parts).

Note   The Goodenough-Harris Drawing Test may be performed in children 5 years or older (see below).

Goodenough-Harris draw-a-man test

Method   This test consists of three sections: (a) draw a man; (b) draw a woman; (c) draw yourself. The test is performed as in 'Draws man with all features'. It is common to ask the child if he has finished before marking a score.

Pass   A scoring system and test results checking table for (a) and (b) are given below. It is a difficult test to score owing to the very detailed scoring system. One point is given for each detail drawn as follows:

1 Head
2 Neck
3 Neck, two dimensions
4 Eyes
5 Eye details: eye brow or lashes
6 Eye detail: pupil
7 Nose
8 Nose, two dimensions
9 Mouth
10 Lips, two dimensions
11 Nose and lips, both in two dimensions
12 Chin and forehead
13 Bridge of nose (straight to eyes, narrower than base)
14 Hair I (any scribble)
15 Hair II (more detail)
16 Ears
17 Fingers
18 Correct number of fingers
19 Opposition of thumb (must include fingers)
20 Hands
21 Arms
22 Arm at side or engaged in activity
23 Feet (any indication)
24 Attachment of arms and legs I (anywhere to trunk)
25 Attachment of arms and legs II (at correct position of trunk)
26 Trunk
27 Trunk in proportion, two dimensions (length greater than breadth)
28 Clothing I (anything)
29 Clothing II (2 articles of clothing)

Goodenough-Harris draw-a-woman test

This test may also be performed. One point is given for each detail drawn as follows:

1 Head
2 Neck
3 Neck, two dimensions
4 Eyes
5 Eye details: eye brow or lashes
6 Eye detail: pupil
7 Nose
8 Nose, two dimensions
9 Nostrils
10 Bridge of nose (straight to eyes, narrower than base)
11 Mouth
12 Lips, two dimensions
13 Nose and lips, both in two dimensions
14 Chin and forehead
15 Hair I (any scribble)
16 Hair II (more detailed)
17 Necklace or ear-ring
18 Finger
19 Correct number of fingers
20 Opposition of thumb (must include fingers)
21 Hands
22 Arms
23 Legs
24 Feet (any indication)
25 Shoe (must be 'feminine' — high heels, open toe, strap, etc)
26 Attachment of arms and legs I (anywhere to trunk)
27 Attachment of arms and legs II (correct point of trunk)
28 Clothing (any)
29 Sleeve
30 Neckline (any indication)
31 Trunk
32 Trunk in proportion, two dimensions

Test results checking table:

	Draw-a-man Test Score		Draw-a-woman Test Score	
Age	By boys	By girls	By boys	By girls
3	4	5	4	6
4	7	7	7	8
5	11	12	11	14
6	13	14	13	16
7	16	17	16	19
8	18	20	20	23

Copies 3 steps from 6 bricks (Pass by examination)

Method The examiner makes 3 steps from 6 bricks without the child seeing how to make the steps. The child is asked to copy.

Pass The child is able to copy.

HEARING AND SPEECH

Speaks fluently and clearly (Pass by history)

Method Ask parents if the child speaks well and is grammatically correct.

Pass Parents say he does. Observe and assess the child.

Note This is only a very crude screening test since almost every adult makes grammatical errors. It is more important to find out whether the child speaks fluently; if the child speaks well at 4 years, it is unlikely that he has a congenital hearing defect. However, children who came from families where other languages are spoken and whose mother tongue is not English may make many mistakes. If speech is inadequate or unclear (because of poor articulation, or omission or substitution of consonants) full assessment is mandatory.

If in doubt, check: (a) comprehension — ask the child: 'What do you do when you are cold?', '. . . hungry?', '. . . tired?' (pass if he answers correctly 2 out of 3); (b) comprehension of prepositions — ask the child: 'Put the brick on the table', '. . . under the table', '. . . in front of the chair', '. . . behind the chair'. Do not help by pointing, moving head or eyes (pass if 3 out of 4 answers are correct). (c) Opposite analogues — ask the child: 'If fire is hot, ice is . . .?', 'Mother is a woman, father is a . . .?', 'An elephant is big, a mouse is . . .?' (pass if 2 out of 3 answers are correct). (d) Definition of words — ask the child: 'What is a ball?', '. . . lake?', '. . . desk?', '. . . house?', '. . . banana?', '. . . curtain?', '. . . ceiling?', '. . . hedge?', '. . . pavement?' (pass if defined in terms of use, shape, what it is made of, or general category, provided 6 out of 8 answers are correct). These are Denver Screening Tests, but other tests may be used, e.g. Griffiths' Test, Reynell Developmental Language Scale.

Some children, especially boys who are left handed, have a family tendency to manifest delay in language development. However, all children whose speech is difficult to understand at 4 years should be referred for full assessment.

Hearing test — audiometry (Pass by examination)

Method   See p.85.

Comforts friends in distress (Pass by history)

Method   Ask parents if the child cares for and comforts a friend who has had a minor accident or is upset about something.

Pass   Parents say he does.

Note   Although it is common at this age for a child to show sympathy, it does depend a great deal on the child's personality as well as his developmental stage.

Chooses own friends (Pass by history)

Method   Ask parents if the child chooses who to play with and to spend a lot of time with.

Pass   Parents say he does.

Note   Further questions about the child's social life may help in assessing the developmental history. Pay attention to whether the child chooses younger or older friends, as this may give a clue to the intellectual and emotional stages of development.

Dramatic group play (Pass by history)

Method   Ask parents if the child joins in plays at school, and if he acts out a role during ordinary play activities with his friends.

Pass   Parents say he does join in acting and make-believe group play.

Note   Some children seem to be actors from birth, whereas others are very shy. Take this into account when assessing parents' answer.

3 VISUAL SCREENING TESTS

Screening of vision and examination of the eye are important for the detection of conditions that interfere with a normal visual image which may lead to permanent visual impairment in children. As children learn by seeing objects and faces, good vision is important.

Visual screening is important for two reasons:

1 Decreased visual acuity (poor eyesight) may lead to inadequate school performance.
2 Disorders of the eyes, and systemic diseases with ocular manifestations, may be identified by an eye examination (e.g. cataract and retinal abnormalities such as choroiditis or retrolental fibroplasia, retinoblastoma, glaucoma and eye muscle imbalance which leads to squint).

Children at risk for visual problems have a full visual screening and eye examination at 6–8 months. The 'at-risk' factors are:

1 Pre-term: risk of retrolental fibroplasia, particularly in those at 28–30 weeks or less.
2 Extremely small for dates: risk of choroiditis (if due to congenital infections).
3 Those with a family history (parents or siblings) of eye problems such as congenital cataract, retinoblastoma, and those with a genetic disorder which has eye involvement.
4 Those with a family history (parents or siblings) of squint or having glasses from childhood.

The following might suggest that the child's vision is poor:

(a) if the child does not fix on the face of the mother (or anyone else) while feeding at 6 weeks;
(b) if the child's eye wanders about from one corner of the eye to the other (while the child is awake and happy) after 6 weeks;
(c) if a white spot is seen in the pupil at any age — cataract could be the cause;
(d) if the child, at any age, holds objects very close to his face when trying to read or look at them carefully;

(e) if the child has a squint in one of his eyes after 6 months
of age — until 6 months, squint on its own does not
usually require referral, provided that the child can
follow objects and does not have wandering eye
movements.

It should be noted that if there is a strong family history of eye
problems, advice from an ophthalmologist or orthoptist is
indicated.

Visual screening tests are performed to detect eye ·
problems early. The key ages for testing are as follows:

1 *At birth.* Within a few days of birth all babies are given a
full examination. This includes looking at the eyes,
especially for cataract and wandering eye movements (a
good torch-light might be necessary if the lighting in the
room is poor).

2 *6 weeks.* The baby should start at faces, especially his
mother's face, while feeding, turn his eyes towards diffuse
light if he is left in a room while awake, and should be able
to fix and follow a bright object. It is best to use a colourful
toy, such as a woollen ball, and move it 90° to either side of
the eye. The child will not follow the object when it
disappears behind his head and reappears on the other side
until later, at 8 months of age.

3 *8 months.*

(a) Near vision is assessed by the ability of the child to fix
on small objects, e.g. a Smartie or a raisin. Silver balls
and 'hundreds and thousands' (cake decorations) can
also be used if the child is able to fix on the larger
objects. At 6 months, fixing vision on a Smartie or
raisin (size 3–4 mm) is suggestive of adequate vision.
Children fix well on small decorations such as hundreds
and thousands, which are 1 mm in size, only at about
10 months.

(b) Distant vision is assessed by the ability of the child to
fix on a small object at 3 m. Place a Smartie at 3 m in
front of the child and ask the child to get it (if he
crawls) or watch to see if the child can see the Smartie.
Repeat the test several times if there is doubt.

(c) Following-the-object response. The child should be
able to follow a toy (woollen ball) around when it is
held away from him at his arm's length. The toy is
moved from the centre all round the circle so that the
child will follow it. At 8 months, the child will follow up
to 90°, look for it on the other side and then follow it
through to mid-line. At this age, the child will look for
a fallen toy. Thus one should drop the toy and watch
the child's reactions. If he looks in the direction of the
fallen toy, the response is satisfactory.

(d) Examination of red reflex (see p.79) to exclude cataract.

(e) Examination for squint (see p.77).

4 *2½–3 years*

(a) Distant vision is assessed by the Sheridan-Gardiner or Developkit (or similar) 5-letter (or picture) test with Key card at 3 m (see below). At 2½ years, a child might refuse to do this test, in which case repeat the test recommended for 8 months.

(b) Near vision is assessed by the ability of the child to fix on 'hundreds and thousands', or by Snellen's near-vision letter type test, with the Key card at a comfortable distance from the child, usually at 0.33 m (see p.73).

5 *4½–5 years*

(a) Distant vision is assessed by the Sheridan-Gardiner or Developkit 5-letter (or picture) test, with or without a Key card at 6 m (or at 3 m) using appropriate letters.

(b) Near vision is assessed by Snellen's letter type test, with or without a Key card at 0.33 m.

TEST FOR DISTANT VISION

Sheridan-Gardiner or Developkit 5-letter (or picture) test with Key card (Pass by examination)

Method

Sit the child on a chair at a small table and place the 5-letter Key card in front of him. The card contains the letters V, H, O, X and T. They are also in a chart (or book) held by the examiner, who should stand at a measured distance from the child. It is best to stand at 6 m, but it is permissible to stand at 3 m, if the room is not long enough. In that case, the letters of appropriate size should be used (use the letters in the 3 m distance vision test chart).

If the child has normal vision at this distance, it should be 3/3, which is equivalent to 6/6. The 6 m test may not work for young children (about 3 years of age) because the examiner will seem to be too far away. Another technique is to use a mirror 3 m from the child, so that the examiner can stand alongside the child and can also see the letters that the child is pointing to. All the letters in the book are symmetrical and therefore can be used with a mirror.

It is useful to have a cord knotted at one end, and with other knots at 3 m and 6 m; the child can be asked to hold one end and the examiner the other to ensure that they are at a correct distance from one another.

The child is best seated at a table; if he holds the Key card he may tip it towards himself and the examiner cannot see whether he is pointing to the right letter or not. A parent or another observer has to sit alongside the child to verify his reaction.

Each eye must be tested independently. There are several methods of achieving this. One can ask a parent to cover each of the child's eyes in turn, or use something to cover each eye. Some authors have recommended a wooden spoon or an eye-patch. The problem is that many young children do not like this method of obstructing their vision and may become unco-operative, so that the test cannot be completed. A better method is to use a pair of children's sunglasses. One lens is covered with opaque strapping and the other lens removed from the frame. With two pairs of such spectacles it is possible to test each eye easily. The children seem to enjoy the 'special' glasses.

The examiner starts by showing the child a letter at close range, and asking him to point to the corresponding letter on the Key card; this is to be sure that the child knows what he is required to do, the examiner then goes to 3 m or 6 m and gradually presents smaller and smaller letters until the child can no longer identify them. The last complete line (2 out of 3 letters) he reads indicates his visual acuity (VA). If it was the right eye which was tested, the results are recorded as VAR (visual acuity right) 6/12, where 6 indicates the distance in metres from the test letters. The other number indicates the distance at which a normal eye can see at 6 m. VA of 6/12 (or 3/6) or less is an indication for referral for ophthal-mological opinion. In addition, a difference of more than one line of letters between each eye's performance is a cause for referral. The test should be done with distance spectacles if the child uses them; this should be stated.

Pin-hole test

A child with a refractive error will improve his VA by 1 or 2 lines, whereas those without will not show any improvement. This is because while looking through a pin-hole the patient's own lens system is not used.

Method   A hole is made with a thick pin on a piece of thin cardboard and the child is asked to look through it. The VA distant-vision test (Sheriden-Gardiner or Developkit 5-letter (or picture) test) is repeated.

Note The single letter method is described above. However, it is best to do the test using the crowded letter method (as in Developkit), in which a group of letters is used. This is more difficult, but it reflects the child's ability to read letters when presented in multiples.

TEST FOR NEAR VISION

Snellen's letter type test (Pass by examination)

Method The child is asked to read (or point to, using the Key card) the letters on the near-vision test (e.g. Reduced Snellen) card, starting from the top to the bottom and going as far down as he can correctly identify them. The distance is usually 0.33 m.

Pass The child is able to read small letters up to N5 or 6/6 (which is the smallest size of newspaper print).

Note If the child wears spectacles the test should be done with and without them and recorded accordingly. There are various cards now available, all of which are almost identical; if the child can read small newspaper print letters, this is adequate. In older children each eye can be tested separately, but in younger children both eyes are tested together.

TEST FOR COLOUR VISION

Several months are available for screening for colour vision; the Ishihara plates (found in *Test for colour-blindness* by Shinobu Ishihara, published by Kanehara Shuppan Co Ltd, Tokyo, Japan) or the Guy's Hospital *Colour vision chart book* are the most commonly used. These tests contain specific colour cards, the so-called pseudo-isochromatic cards. A person with normal colour vision should be able to read all the numbers (in the Ishihara book) or letters (in the Guy's book) without mistakes. Persons with defective colour vision will make mistakes.

Method Ask the child to read all the numbers (or letters) in one of the colour-vision test books. The room should have adequate lighting, but should not be in direct sunlight because the shadows can interfere with the test. The plates are held 75 cm (2½ feet) from the child and tilted so that the plane of the paper is at right angles to the line of vision.

Pass The child reads the first number (or letter) correctly. The correct answer is found in the book. If the child did not read the first letter correctly (which is number 12 in the Ishihara book), then he is unable to understand the test or his vision is poor. Colour-vision testing is then not possible.

The numbers which are seen by the child (and stated) should be recorded. The child should give the answers without more than 3 s delay. For those who cannot read, the numbers may be traced with the index finger (the examiner should record the number the child has indicated).

Check the answers given by the child against the correct answers in the book. If the child has made mistakes and read it differently, then colour-vision abnormality is present. The answer sheet also shows how people with red-green deficiencies and those with total colour blindness and weakness will read a test; this gives a quick and accurate assessment of colour-vision deficiency of congenital origin, which is the commonest form of colour disturbance.

Most children with congenital colour-vision deficiency are characterized by a red-green deficiency which may be of two types; first, a protan type which may be absolute (protanopia) or partial (protanomalopia), and secondly, a deutan type which may be absolute (deuteranopia) or partial (deuteranomalopia).

In protanopia, the visible range of the spectrum is shorter at the red end compared with that of normal vision, and that part of the spectrum which appears to the normal vision as blue-green appears to those with protanopia as grey. The whole visible range of the spectrum in protanopia consists of two areas, which are separated from one another by this grey part. Each area appears to those with protanopia as one system of colour with different brightness and saturation within each area, the colour in one area being different from that of the other. The red with a slight tinge of purple, which is the complementary colour of blue-green, appears as grey.

In duteranopia, that part of the spectrum which appears to the normal vision as green, appears as grey, and the visible range of the spectrum is divided by these zones into two areas, each of which appears to be of one colour system. The visible range of the spectrum is not contracted, in contrast to protanopia, Purple-red, which is the complementary colour of green, appears also as grey.

In protanomalopia and deuteranomalopia, there is no part of the spectrum which appears grey, but the part of the spectrum which appears to those with protanopia as grey appears to those with protanomalia as a greyish indistinct colour, and likewise, the grey part of the spectrum seen by the person with deuteranopia appears to those with deuteranomalopia as an indistinct colour close to grey.

Consequently, one of the peculiarities of red-green deficiencies is that blue and yellow colours appear to be remarkably clear compared with red and green colours. The application of this peculiarity to the test for colour-vision deficiency is the distinguishing feature of the Ishihara test.

In the very rare congenital colour-vision deficiencies, there is total colour weakness. The colour sensitivity of the total weakness to red-green, as well as to yellow and blue, is very low and only the clear colours can be perceived; but, except for the colour sensitivity, there is no abnormality in the visual functions. The plates in Ishihara's book form an easy method of establishing the diagnosis in such cases and of distinguishing them from cases of red-green deficiency.

There is also a very rare group of persons who suffer from total colour blindness and show a complete failure to discriminate any colour variations, usually with an associated impairment of central vision with photophobia and nystagmus.

Finally, a failure of the appreciation of blue and yellow is termed tritanomalopia if partial, and tritanopia if absolute. Such cases are extremely rare and the plates in Ishihara's book are not designed for their diagnosis.

NOTES ON COLOUR VISION

Colour-vision deficiency is common in boys (sex-linked recessive). It probably occurs in ratios of about 1:10 for boys and in 1:250 for girls.

Red-green colour blindness is the commonest. However, partial deficiency is more common than total deficiency. For practical purposes, these persons are normal.

Pathophysiology

There is a deficiency of pigments in the retinal cone cells. The absence of pigments gives total colour blindness.

Clinical features

Clinical features are not usually apparent. However, since colour discrimination is poor, especially under poor lighting conditions, these persons are not able to do jobs where colour discrimination is essential. This includes working in the printing and dyeing industries. These individuals are not taken as pilots, train drivers, or in the army and police forces. They are excluded from electrical engineering apprenticeships.

Employment

Guidance is required for those affected. Those with partial deficiency are treated normally. Help from an employment adviser may be sought.

Treatment

There is no treatment, but early advice on careers can be given to discourage those affected from training for unsuitable occupations. There are those who question whether screening for colour vision should be continued, since there is little benefit for those affected and there is no effective therapy. However, part of child health surveillance is giving advice on various health matters, education and employment and consequently this screening will probably have to be continued.

TESTS FOR SQUINT

Hirschberg corneal light reflection test

Method Sit the child comfortably on a parent's lap or in a chair. The examiner faces the child and stands in front of him. He then, without warning, shines a bright light from a pen-torch or ophthalmoscope at 50 cm (approximately an arm's length) from the child. He should attract the child's attention to the light, initially fixing the child's head in the mid-line with one hand (Fig. 41). The examiner can also look for the reflections of light from a distant window, thus avoiding the use of a light source.

Pass Reflection of the light on the cornea of each eye is symmetrical, near the centre of the pupil — it is usual for the reflections to be slightly towards the nose (Fig. 42a–c).

Now turn the child's head to one side and watch for the corneal reflections while the fixation is maintained. The corneal reflex should remain symmetrical. Repeat the test by turning the head to the other side (in an older child, the light source could be moved to the right and then to the left while the child is fixing to the light source).

Note If reflections are not symmetrical (Fig. 42d), strabismus may be present and a cover test should be done. Ask parents if they have noticed a squint.

Pseudosquints, due to epicanthic folds, are often mistaken as squint by parents, but corneal light reflections in these children are symmetrical (Fig. 42a, e).

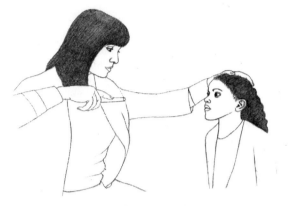

Fig. 41 Hirschberg corneal light reflection test

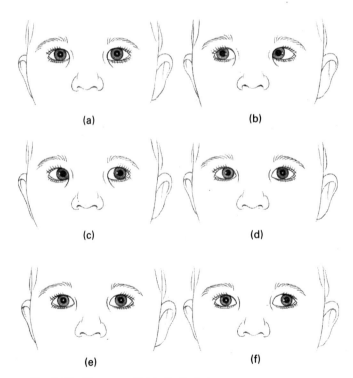

Fig. 42 Hirschberg corneal light reflection test

Cover test (Fig. 43a–c)

Method   The child sits comfortably on a parent's lap or in a chair. The
examiner faces the child and stands in front of him. He then,
without warning, shines a bright light from a torch or
ophthalmoscope (as in Hirschberg's test) at 50 cm from the
child. It is probably best to use a small bright object and ask
child to look at it. Attract the child's attention and while he is
watching the light or object, one of his eyes is covered by the
examiner's hand or using a card (eye must be fully covered).

Pass   Watch for any movement of the uncovered eye to fix on the
light/object. Then remove the cover and watch the covered
eye to see if it moves to fix on the light/object. Repeat the
same test with the other eye. The test is positive if the eyes
deviate (move) to fix either when covered or when the cover
is removed (the uncover test). Thus, if either or both eyes
move, a squint is present.

Left convergent squint — eyes in the primary position. A left
convergent squint is shown in Figure 43(a) — note the
asymmetry of the corneal light reflex. When the right eye is
covered, the left eye moves out to take up fixation (Fig. 43b).
When the cover is removed the left eye moves in again to the
primary position (Fig. 43a).

*Alternating left convergent squint — eyes in the primary
position.* When the right eye is covered, the left eye moves

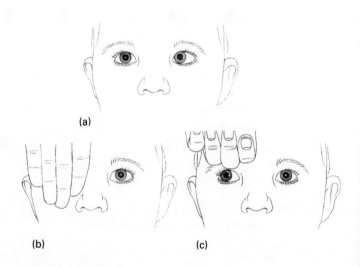

(a)

(b)   (c)

Fig. 43 Cover test

out to take up fixation (Fig. 43b). When the cover is removed, the left eye *does not move* in again but remains straight (Fig. 43c). The right eye now remains convergent, i.e. right convergent squint.

Unilateral squint. This is when the squinting eye takes up fixation when the other eye is covered, but returns to the squinting position as soon as the cover is removed.

Alternating squint. This is when the squinting eyes take up fixation when the other eye is covered, but retains fixation even when the cover is removed, with the previously fixing eye remaining in the deviated position.

Latent squint. This is when the squint is not manifest all the time, but only at times of stress or when the child is tired or ill. Rapid cover test will demonstrate this, but a slow cover test may miss it. Therefore, if the parents have noticed a squint it could be a latent squint and this should be looked for.

Brueckner red reflex test

Method   Sit the child comfortably on a parent's lap or in a chair. The examiner faces the child and stands in front of him. If possible the room light should be dimmed (to decrease the child's interest in other stimuli in the room and for better contrast). The examiner should direct the ophthalmoscope beam at 50 cm (1½ feet) from the base of the child's nose, using the large white spot on the target wheel. Both eyes should be encompassed by the beam of light. The examiner should now look through the ophthalmoscope and get a clear view of the child's cornea (Fig. 44). To do this, the examiner may have to turn the focusing wheel to +2 or +3.

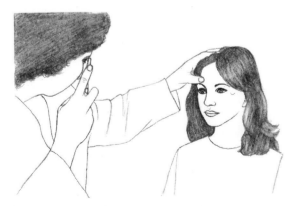

Fig. 44 Brueckner red reflex test

Pass   The bright red reflex (from the retina) should be seen clearly and in the non-squinting eye it should be symmetrical and identical in colour; it should fill both pupils entirely. The colour may vary slightly from the top of the pupil to the bottom — from a tinge of yellow to bright red. When a squint is present, only one eye at a time looks directly at the light from the ophthalmoscope. The fixing eye will thus have a darker red reflex and a slightly smaller pupil (due to pupillary reflex). The squinting eye will have a more orange-red reflex and larger pupil (Fig. 45).

Note   A positive Brueckner test (i.e. when asymmetry is present) indicates the possibility of a squint. However, there are two other causes for a positive test: mild cataract and corneal scarring, both of which need a fundal examination (after pupillary dilatation) for clear differentiation.

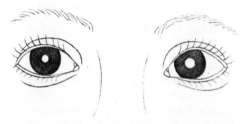

Fig. 45 Brueckner test. Red reflexes and corneal light reflexes are asymmetrical. The non-fixing eye has a larger pupil than the fixing eye. The child has left convergent squint.

4 HEARING SCREENING TESTS

TESTS FROM BIRTH TO 6 WEEKS

Startle response (Pass by examination or history)

Method   Clap suddenly at 30 cm (1 foot) or ask parents if they think the child can hear, for example, a sudden noise, such as the door being shut in another room or the telephone ringing.

Pass   The child stiffens, blinks, screws up eyes, extends limbs or cries.

Note   This is a crude test, but helpful. Startling by noise indicates that the child can hear, but since loud noise (60–70 dB) is used for this test, it will detect severe hearing loss. Therefore, it is important to remember that moderate hearing loss will be missed by this screening method.

Rattle or bell (Pass by examination)

Method   Hold a rattle or bell so that the child cannot see it. Sound it quietly for 3–5 s at 15 cm (6 inches) at ear level, with 5 s pauses. Increase loudness if there is no response.

Pass   The child quietens in response to this sound. The commonest response is turning or widening of the eyes or a change in breathing pattern.

Note   If the child does not respond, try again after a short while. If he does not show any response, repeat again after 2 weeks. Ask the parents if the baby can hear. If the parents do not think the child can hear, ask them to observe and to return in about 2 weeks' time.

The limitation of this screening test is also that it can detect only severe hearing loss. The noise made by the bell (or rattle) is about 50 dB; therefore, hearing loss below this will be missed. Nevertheless, it is important to notice severe loss at this age, so this method of screening is still useful.

If a child consistently does not respond to any of the above two tests at 6 weeks, referral to an audiologist is important.

Infant screening audiometers

These are not widely available and are *not* recommended (at present) as a routine neonatal hearing screening test. These are various models and types available.

Method   Present an auditory stimulus to each of the infant's ears separately by the audiometer. The noise may be given by a cradle worn by the baby or by holding the instrument at 15 cm (6 inches) at ear level as he lies in the cot (different instruments have different types of sound delivery system). Make noise for 2 s.

Pass   Responds by stilling, eye widening, eye-blinking, grimacing or by sucking reflex, or change in the breathing pattern. Stilling or blinking is the usual response. Test is best done 1 h before feeding. The responses can be recorded and analysed by computer.

Note   Failure on 2 separate occasions, 1 week apart, has the same significance as in the rattle or bell test.

At present these are experimental apparatuses and are expensive. False positive and false negative results occur, mainly due to observer error. The advantages of early (in the newborn period) detection and treatment of severe hearing loss, as opposed to detection at 3–4 months, is not clear. However, there are advantages in detecting it by 3 months (but not earlier), so that a hearing-aid may be given and parents may be trained to speak to the child.
Practical points. Do not label the child deaf until absolutely sure. Prepare parents slowly for diagnosis and management — it helps with bonding.

TESTS AT 8 TO 12 MONTHS

The best age for hearing screening test is 8–10 months and not before 6 months (the brain is not 'mature' enough) or after 15 months (the child is difficult to distract). By 8 months the child is sensitive to sound, is able to sit well and has very good head control. In addition, he will turn his head to locate sound.

Distraction hearing test (Pass by examination)

This test was described by Sir Alexander and Lady Irene Ewing at the University of Manchester, UK. An assistant is required to distract the child, which is why the method is known as 'distraction testing'. A visually alert child may get visual clues and respond to them, giving false positive results. False negative results may be due to middle ear dysfunction (which accounts from 20–30 dB loss), wax or if the infant is tired, hungry or non-specifically unwell. The room may be noisy (background noise should be minimal during testing). The tester uses various standardised sounds and test materials:

1 *Manchester rattle*. Produces low-frequency sounds (about 4000 Hz).
2 *Nuffield rattle*. Produces high-frequency sounds (up to about 8000 Hz) and is therefore a good test instrument for high-tone hearing. It produces sound equal in loudness to the 'ss' and 'sh' sounds in normal conversational speech.
3 *Arousal sounds*. (a) Rustling paper (not widely used now) — high frequency; (b) bell (also not widely used now) — high frequency; (c) cup with a spoon — high frequency.
4 *Voice*. (a) whisper child's name (soft whisper is 40 dB), 'Hello John, look what I have got', 'Look here John', 'Mary, can you hear me' — low frequency; (b) 'Oo-oo' (as in 'boo' or 'poo') — low frequency; (c) 'ss' (as in bus, not 'sh' or 'z') — high frequency); (d) 'pth-pth' (not widely used now) — high frequency.

Method   See page 27 for full description and interpretation.

Pass   From 6 months onwards, the child is able to localise sound; by 8 months, responses must be good.

Localisation is searching for and finding a source of sound, not at ear level, but above or below the ear:

1 *By 6 months*. The child turns his eyes laterally and then to the source of sound. He turns his eyes to the direction of the sound and then below ear level (see Figs 16a and 16b on p.27).
2 *By 7 months*. The child can do this by a smooth arc, i.e. he turns his eyes to the direction of sound and then turns his head by a smooth arc.
3 *By 8 months*. The child can locate in a straight line.

Note   Inferior localisation (looking for sound source below) occurs before superior.

TESTS FOR THE OLDER CHILDREN (2–5 YEARS)

Two games used for testing are (a) go-game, and (b) the speech discrimination test. In children with mental subnormality and who are unco-operative, other methods of testing may have to be used, e.g. 'free-field' testing.

Audiometry is possible by 3 years — it needs co-operation and understanding. It should be done if other tests are failed or doubtful response is obtained.

Stycar hearing tests for older children are also popular but need special training. Details are given in *Manual for the Stycar hearing tests* by Mary D Sheridan. This book is supplied with special test equipment box. It gives different tests at different age groups.

The following screening tests are more popular:

Go-game

This test is useful for children aged 2–4 years and for children with mental subnormality functioning at the 3–4-year-old level. The child's co-operation and understanding are required.

Method   Ask the child to drop a brick into a box when he hears the word 'go' (first train him a few times). The test may be done using plastic cups and the child is asked to put one cup over the other each time he hears the sound. The examiner's mouth should be covered and the word 'go' said more and more softly. An experienced tester can drop the voice to below 40 dB.

Pass   The child does the game properly and drops the brick or puts the cups over each other in response to the command.

Note   Failure has the same significance as failing the hearing test at 6–8 months — the same procedure is to be adopted (see p.27).

Speech discrimination test

This test is useful for children aged 2 years and over and for mentally retarded children with 2-year-old comprehension. The child's co-operation and understanding are required. This test is more difficult than the go-game.

Method   See page 47.

'Free-field' testing

This test may be used until pure tone audiometry is reliably possible (at age 4 years and/or 6–10 years for children with mild/moderate mental subnormality, depending on severity). It is done without earphones; sounds are produced at some distance from the ears. The frequency of sounds is in the range 250–8000 Hz. The frequency of sounds (in Hz) produced by various instruments is as follows:

Xylophone: 250, 500, 1000, 2000, 4000
Pitch pipes: 250, 500, 750, 1000, 2000, 4000
Tuning fork: 125, 250, 500, 1000, 2000, 4000

Method   Observe the child at play and his reactions to sounds in the free field. Make various sounds (using xylophone, pitch pipes, tuning form) and talk — intensity may be measured by a sound-level meter.

Pass   The assessment made by observation of reactions to sound is satisfactory (this excludes significant deafness, and confirms that hearing is adequate for speech).

Note   If failed, try pure-tone audiometry; if not possible, significant hearing loss is possible. Begin hearing-aid training and try audiometry later. Alternatively, auditory-evoked responses may be arranged.

Pure-tone audiometry (Pass by examination)

Audiometry measures the ability to hear pure tones which are produced by the audiometer. The intensity (measured in decibels) and frequency (measured in Hertz) are adjustable so that the audiometery can deliver sounds. The sounds can be delivered by earphone to test air conduction and by headband to the mastoid to test bone conduction.

Method   The child puts on the headphone which should be placed centrally covering the auditory meatus (ears). The '10 down–5 up' technique is used.

1 All pure tones are presented at 1–3 s separated by 1–3 s. It is important to avoid any rhythm, so that the child cannot guess in anticipation.

2 Start at 1000 Hz and increase to 2000, 4000, 8000 Hz. Then check at 250 and 500 Hz. It is customary to present the initial sound at 40 dB, at 1000 Hz. If the child hears this, the sound level is reduced by 10 dB until he ceases to hear. Then increase the sound level in steps of 5 dB until he can hear. This gives the child's hearing threshold level.

This method takes at least 10 min to perform and therefore a screening method is often employed. This is the sweep audiometry.

Sweep audiometry

This method is employed for testing large numbers of children, and it is often performed at the pre-school entry examination or in the first year at the infant school and in the first year at the junior school. It is often done by a specialist trained nurse.

Using a pure-tone audiometry, various ranges of frequencies are tested at a fixed intensity level (often at 25 dB). The child is presented with sounds at 2000, 4000, 8000 and then 250, 500 and 1000 Hz. Each ear is tested separately.

If the child fails to hear in any one frequency, it is taken as failure and a full audiological screening using a pure-tone audiometer is important.

5 GENERAL EXAMINATION

EXAMINATION OF TESTICLES

Testicles should be routinely examined in all boys. At birth, a full-term boy should have descended testicles, although they may still be in the groin or abdomen in a pre-term baby. If the testicles have descended fully into the scrotum, this should be recorded in the notes. There is no further need to worry about their descent, even though they may retract. In middle childhood, retraction is very common and it may be difficult to draw the testicles down into the scrotum. A useful manoeuvre is to ask the boy to squat on a chair. The cremaster muscles will then relax and the testicles should drop naturally into the scrotum.

Method The infant lies on his back and the examiner palpates the scrotum for the testicles. Each side is palpated separately. (The hands of the examiner should *not* be cold.)

Note If a testicle has not descended at birth, it is usual to examine it again at 3 months or later. Referral to a surgeon should be considered by 1 year of age if the testicle has still not descended. A bilateral undescended testicle should be an indication for a general assessment and possibly a chromosome analysis.

EXAMINATION OF HIPS

Hips should be examined at birth, 6 weeks, 6–8 months and in the second year (15–21 months of age).

Note   Congenital dislocation of the hip encompasses varying degrees of instability, subluxation and dysplasia of the hip joint and should no longer be regarded in terms of simple 'dislocation'. The term is therefore inaccurate, strictly speaking, but is being retained because of its long-standing usage.

Congenital dislocation of the hip (CDH) is defined as: 'A congenital deformation of the hip joint in which the head of the femur is, or may be, partially or completely displaced from the acetabulum. The term embraces secondary hip dysplasia whether or not hip instability or dislocation persist.'

In the newborn baby, limited abduction is uncommon as a sign of dislocated hip. It is seen sometimes in babies with neurological abnormalities, such as spina bifida, where a fixed dislocation has developed before birth. It is important to be very cautious while abducting the hip, because it is possible to fracture the femur if too much strain is put on the bone when the hip is flexed. In early weeks of life, the most important sign of CDH is instability of the hip.

TESTS FOR CDH: FROM NEWBORN PERIOD UP TO 3 MONTHS

The baby lies on his back with his legs towards examiner and the hips abducted and fully flexed. At this age, the femur is gently abducted at the hip. This should be done on each side. The pelvis is held steady by grasping the other femur between the thumb and the fingers. The thumb is held on the symphysis pubis and the fingers are under the sacrum. The other hand is then used to abduct the hip gently. One thigh is grasped by the examiner's hand, with the middle finger over the greater trochanter — the flexed leg is held in the palm, with the thumb on the inner side of the thigh opposite the lesser trochanter. When the hip is dislocated, it will slip back into joint and the femoral head is felt to move (0.5 cm). During this manouevre a sudden jump, jab or judder is felt as the head of the femur slips into the cup on the pelvis which is known as the acetabulum. The left hip is more commonly dislocated but both hips must be tested independently. This manipulation is often known as the Ortolani manoeuvre (Fig. 46).

If the hips are not dislocated, the next test is to see if they are dislocatable. Again the pelvis is steadied by one hand. The other is used to move the femoral head forward into, and backwards out of, the acetabulum. The purpose is to see if the head of the femur can be pushed over the rim of the acetabulum. The manoeuvre is rather like following the head of the femur between the thumb and first two fingers. When the hip is dislocated, the judder of the femoral head slipping in and out of the joint can be felt easily, with a movement of not more than 0.5 cm. This is the Barlow manoeuvre (Fig. 47).

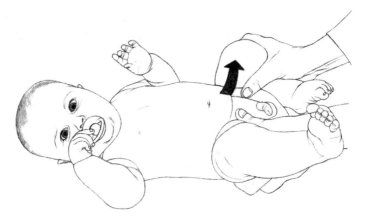

Fig. 46 Ortolani manoeuvre

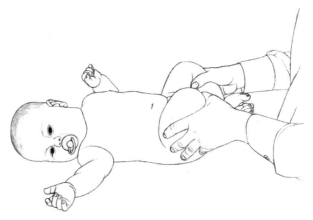

Fig. 47 Barlow manoeuvre

The two tests should also be performed together, and this is then known as the modified Ortolani-Barlow manoeuvre (Fig. 48).

Some people refer to clicks in the hip joint (without movement). These do not indicate a dislocation or a dislocatable joint. The sensation obtained from a dislocated joint is often described as a 'clunk' and not a 'click'. When a click is heard or felt, it is important to establish whether it comes from the hip or another place, usually the knee. There is some suggestion that a click in the hip needs a careful follow-up because of the increased risk later of hip abnormalities, but the significance is not nearly as serious as a clunk. It is better to use the term 'ligamentous click', since Ortolani's description in Italian of a judder has been mistranslated into English as a click. Ligamentous clicks, without movement of the head of the femur, are elicitable in 5–10% of babies, and they are of no clinical significance.

TEST FOR CDH: 6–8 MONTHS, 1 YEAR AND 18 MONTHS

Examination of the hip after the first few weeks of life is a little different. It is then unusual, but still possible (even up to 2 years), to elicit the sign often described as a clunk. The Ortolani manoeuvre is performed and a clunk can be felt as the head of the femur reduces. However, the critical sign is limitation of abduction.

The infant lies on his back with hips flexed at 90°. Any hip which cannot be abducted to 75° must be viewed with suspicion. It is sometimes helpful to place the baby prone, to see how far the legs will abduct.

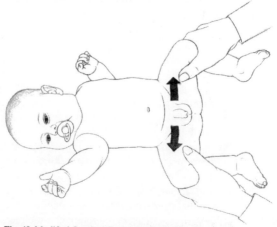

Fig. 48 Modified Ortolani-Barlow manoeuvre

The most useful investigations at present are X-rays and ultrasound. An X-ray can be arranged at 4–6 months of age when the femoral head becomes ossified and its relationship to the acetabulum can be seen. The cartilage in the femoral head at birth can be clearly seen on ultrasound, a technique which is likely to be used more in future; it becomes less useful when bone appears in the femoral head and blocks the sound.

There are, of course, other causes of limitation of abduction in infancy and childhood, one of the most common being increased muscle tone in spasticity.

The following signs of unilateral dislocation should also be looked for:

1 *Leg posture.* The thigh on the affected side tends to be held in partial lateral rotation, flexion and abduction.
2 *Limb shortening.* Above-knee shortening may be apparent when the suspect limb is compared with the normal leg. The level of the knees should be compared.
3 *Asymmetry of thighs.* When the hips are held in flexed position, asymmetry of skin creases to the inside of the thigh may be apparent.
4 *Flattening of the buttock.* In the prone position, the buttock on the side of the dislocation may appear to be flattened.

Notes 1 Hip examinations are done within 24 h of birth and at the time of discharge from the hospital, or at about 10 days of age, but it is not always possible to detect every CDH at that time. Thus, it is important to continue the surveillance at least until the child is seen to be walking normally. The hips should be examined at the developmental check at 8 months.

2 The person who tested the hips for CDH should keep an accurate record, noting when and where the examinations were carried out and recording the results clearly.

3 'At risk' groups for CDH: (a) most common in girls and in first-born babies; (b) family history of CDH; (c) infants presenting by the breech; (d) other congenital posture deformities such as those of the foot; (e) birth by Caesarean section; (f) oligohydramnios; (g) fetal growth of retardation. These children need an extra careful examination.

4 In some children, CDH is not present at birth but may appear much later due to an abnormality in the acetabulum (acetabular dysplasia). This condition is hereditary and shows an autosomal dominant inheritance. Careful examination during infancy will demonstrate such deformity. A first-degree relative of such a child may have hip problems in adulthood.

EXAMINATION FOR SCOLIOSIS

Screening for scoliosis (curvature of the spine) is important because the early onset variety can be progressive. The late onset form (adolescent scoliosis), which occurs during puberty, is not serious; it is mainly a cosmetic problem, but can occasionally cause pain.

The early onset form (before 8 years of age) is not only responsible for severe cosmetic problems, but can cause cardiopulmonary disturbance (lung function impairment due to impaired lung development). The pain can be quite severe.

Thus scoliosis, especially congenital scoliosis, should be found as early as possible — by 6 months to 1 year — since early treatment prevents progression.

Children at risk of developing scoliosis include those with the following problems:

1 Congenital malformations of the spine: butterfly vertebra.
2 Neuromuscular problems, e.g. cerebral palsy, muscular dystrophy, spina bifida, hypotonia from any cause (congenital myopathies, etc), poliomyelitis.
3 Connective tissue disorders: Morphan's syndrome.
4 Others: neurofibromatosis, bone dysplasias, Frederick's ataxia.

Clinical features include: (a) difference in shoulder height; (b) obvious spinal curvature; (c) difference in space between the trunk and the upper limbs.

Note Bending the child over can detect at 5° rotation at the spine. Scoliosis which disappears on bending (but is apparent when straight) is postural scoliosis and is of no clinical significance. Scoliosis with spinal rotation (which is significant) does not disappear on bending. This is structural scoliosis which, if untreated, can cause vertebral rotation (rotation wedging).

In young infants (6 weeks, 8 months, 1 year)

Method Place infant prone (on the tummy) and feel the shoulder and in the thoracic cage. Also look for an apparent hump.

Pass No rib hump or shoulder hump.

Note The presence of a hump indicates scoliosis; the child should be referred for X-ray of the whole spine and for an orthopaedic opinion.

In older children

Method Ask the child to bend forward while he is standing straight with both feet together and holding both hands straight. Look for a shoulder, thoracic or lumbar hump. Also look for difference in shoulder height, obvious spinal curvature and the gap between the arm and waist. Look for asymmetry of the scapula or waistline.

Pass There is no hump or prominence of the rib cage with gibbus; there is no asymmetry of the scapula or gap between the arm and waist.

Note It might be helpful for the examiner to perform a control bending of the child by standing in front of him and watching for scoliosis. Asymmetry of the scapula or waistline may also indicate scoliosis.

A child who has significant scoliosis should be referred for an orthopaedic opinion.

GESSELL, BINET AND BENDER-GESTALT TEST (MODIFIED)

15 months : Scribbles spontaneously
18 months : Imitates stroke
2 years   : Imitates vertical line within 30°
2½ years   : Imitates horizontal line

Note   From the age of 3 years onwards the tests applied are 'copy' and not 'imitate'. In an imitation test, the tester draws the diagram in front of the child and shows how to make it — the child is then asked to 'draw one like this'. In a copy test, the tester draws the diagram without showing how it is drawn, or produces a ready-made diagram and asks the child to copy — 'draw one like this'.

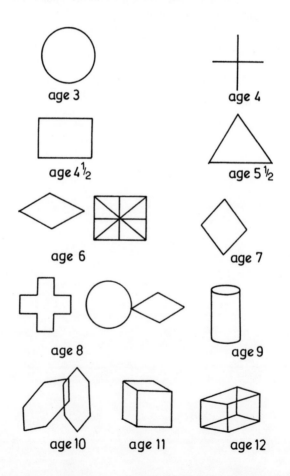

APPENDIX

CHILD

Name: ....   Sex: ....

Address: ....   Clinic/Hospital (No): ....

Date of birth: ....

Category	6 WEEKS	6 MONTHS	8 MONTHS	1 YEAR
SOCIAL BEHAVIOUR AND PLAY **B**	Turns to regard observer's face HE; Smiles HE	Plays 'peek-a-boo' EH; Hand and foot regard HE; Puts everything to mouth HE		Waves goodbye H; Plays 'pat-a-cake' EH; Indicates wants (not by crying) H; Drinks from cup H; Scoliosis; Distraction hearing test E
HEARING AND SPEECH **S**	Scoliosis; Startle response E; Rattle or bell, 15cm at ear level E	Responds to own name H; Laughs H; Vocalizes EH; Distraction hearing test E	Polysyllabic babbling EH; Testicles ***; ***	Understands several words H; Uses 'mama' and 'dada' H; Turns to sound of name HE; ***; Holds 2 bricks and bangs them together E
FINE MOTOR AND VISION **V**	Testicles; Follows horizontally to 90° E; Stares EH; Hips	Follows fallen toys E; Fixes on small objects E; Transfers and mouths EH; Reaches out to grasp (palmar grasp) HE; Hips		Pincer grasp E; Casts HE; Points with index finger H; Hips
GROSS MOTOR **M**	Hips; Prone position E; Ventral suspension E; Moro response E; Head control E	Can be pulled to sit E; Sits with support HE; Bears weight on legs E	Crawls E; Forward parachute response E; Sits without support E; Downward parachute response E; Rolls over from back to prone E	Walks alone EH; Walks holding furniture EH; Pulls to standing position EH; Gets to sitting position EH

USUAL AGE OF ATTAINMENT	6 WEEKS	6 MONTHS	8 MONTHS	1 YEAR
DATE AND AGE				
PRESENT ATTAINMENT	M V S B	M V S B	M V S B	M V S B

**   = Sheridan–Gardiner Near Vision Test, Sheridan–Gardiner Distant Vision Test
*** = Hirschberg Corneal Light Reflection Test; Cover Test

DEVELOPMENT

18 MONTHS	2-2½ YEARS	3 YEARS	4 YEARS	5 YEARS
			Dresses without supervision H	Dramatic group play H
		Separates from mother easily		Chooses own friends H
Indicates toilet needs H	Dry throughout day H	Washes and dries hands HE		Comforts friends in distress H
Takes off shoes and socks H	Puts on clothes H	Dresses with supervision H	Brushes teeth H	
Explores environment	Eats with spoon and fork H	Goes to toilet alone H	Shares toys H	
Holds spoon — gets food to mouth H	Plays alone H	Eats with knife and fork H		Hearing test — E Audiometry
			Scoliosis	
		Gives full name, sex and age EH	Recognises colours EH	
Obeys simple instruction — 'close the door' HE	Hearing test; Speech discrimination test E	Uses sentences of 4 words HE	Gives full name, age and address EH	
Points to eyes, nose and mouth HE	Gives name HE	Uses prepositions HE	Counts up to 10 EH	Speaks fluently and clearly H
Utters 3 or more other words than 'mama' and 'dada' H	Uses plurals HE		Speech grammatically correct E	
Jabbers continually EH				**••
			Draws man with 3 parts E	Copies 3 steps from 6 bricks E
•••	Builds tower of 8 bricks E	**••	Copies bridge of 3 bricks E	Threads beads well E
Builds tower of 3 or 4 bricks E	Imitates vertical line E	Matches 2 colours E		Draws man with all features E
Turns pages H	Picks up 'hundreds and thousands' E	Threads beads well E	Copies cross and square E	Copies triangle E
Scribbles HE		Copies circle E		
Delicate pincer grasp E				Walks backwards E heel-to-toe
		Stands on one foot 1 second E	Walks heel-to-toe E	Bounces and catches ball HE
Climbs on to chair	Kicks ball EH	Pedals tricycle H	Stands on one foot for 5 seconds E	
Climbs stairs H	Jumps in place E	Climbs stairs in adult manner H	Climbs ladder/ tree/slide E	Walks downstairs one foot per step H
Carries toys while walking HE	Climbs and descends stairs H	Runs fast H	Hops on one foot for 2 metres forward E	
Walks backwards HE				

M	V	S	B	M	V	S	B	M	V	S	B	M	V	S	B	M	V	S	B

E = Pass by examination   Hips = Check for dislocation
H = Pass by history   Testicles = Check for presence and descent   *by S. LINGAM, Jan. 1987*

IDENTIFICATION OF HEARING PROBLEMS IN YOUNG CHILDREN

SCREENING BY HEALTH VISITORS

Any of the following maybe due to hearing loss.
In addition to the tests in the "Child Development" chart, the parent
should be asked the following questions. State date and tick box.

	Date	Yes	No
6 weeks 1. Does the baby pause to listen to loud noises, such as the noise from a vacuum cleaner, radio or television			
3/4 months (*During the 1st visit for immunisation*) 2. Does the baby quieten or smile to a sound even if he cannot see the person making the sound			
3. Does the baby turn his head or eyes searching for the sound if the speaker speaks to him from the side			
6/7 months (*During the 2nd visit for immunisation*) 4. Does the baby turn to locate quiet sounds or voices across the room			
9/11 months (*During the 3rd visit for immunisation*) 5. Does the baby take notice of everyday sounds, such as the noise when parents walk into the room, or when the telephone rings.			
15/18 months (*During the visit for measles immunisation*) 6. Does the baby respond to familiar words (dolly, teddy or car)			

**At each visit ask if there is any doubt
about the baby's ability to hear.
(State: Yes or No)**

6w	4m	7m	9m	15m

IDENTIFICATION OF HEARING PROBLEMS IN OLDER CHILDREN

SCREENING BY HEALTH VISITORS

Any of the following may be due to hearing loss.
The parent should be asked the following questions.
It should be filled in at 2½ and 4½ years during the developmental
screening tests. State date and tick box.

Does the child:-	2½ y Date: Yes	No	4½ y Date: Yes	No
1) show a lack of attention when someone is talking especially if the speaker is behind the child				
2) have defective speech				
3) have difficulty in locating a speaker, or ignore a speaker altogether				
4) appear stubborn or shy or show unco-operative or aggressive behaviour which is not consistent				
5) show wild behaviour after a period of concentration requiring listening				
6) show reluctance to listen to stories read from a book				
7) look intently at a speaker				
8) hear the television or radio only when the volume is turned up				

**At each visit ask if there is any doubt
about the child's ability to hear.
(State: Yes or No)**

2½y	4½y

INDEX